IN THE SHADOW OF THE WHITE PLAGUE

Thomas Y. Crowell, Publishers
Established 1834
New York

IN THE SHADOW OF THE WHITE PLAGUE

A Memoir by

Elizabeth Mooney

FIRST EDITION

Designed by Gloria Adelson

Library of Congress Cataloging in Publication Data

Mooney, Elizabeth Comstock.
  In the shadow of the white plague.
    1. Tuberculosis—Biography. 2. Comstock, Bess.
I. Title.
BC312.M66   362.1'9'699509 (B)   78-3311
ISBN 0-690-01696-4

79 80 81 82 83 10 9 8 7 6 5 4 3 2 1

for Booth,
who never knew
but would have loved Bess

Grateful acknowledgment for help in the research of this book is made above all to Bill McLaughlin, who gave generously of his time when I needed it, and to Alice Wareham, whose letters were invaluable. And to Eugene Keough, who is a born oral historian, and to Tony Anderson and Tom Ward.

I am also grateful to Dr. Francis Trudeau, Jr., and his mother, Mrs. Francis Trudeau, and Mrs. H. M. Kinghorn for a look back into the Saranac of yesterday, and to Irving Altman and Kootchie Hale, whose memories were so helpful.
E.M.

IN THE
SHADOW OF
THE WHITE
PLAGUE

❧ Prologue

As with any history, personal or otherwise, there will be those who say of this book, it wasn't like that.

And in some respects perhaps they will be right. What I have written here is how I remember it, impressions that stayed with me, my mother's history as seen through my eyes. As each of us is a slightly different person to everyone who knows us, so undoubtedly my mother will surely have seemed different to any who are still left who remember her.

They are very few. Nor are there many of us still around who remember when tuberculosis was a dread disease, a tragedy that most frequently struck the young. But among those who do, there are bound to be one or two who will complain that some of my dates are wrong, that I have confused the chronology, the personal facts on which my mother's story hangs.

It could well be. I was looking down a tunnel peopled largely with those who have gone. And I was young.

And how did I know what they said in another city fifty years ago when I wasn't even there? They told me, when it was all over and it didn't matter anymore. There is something in all of us that wants to set the record straight, pass on what we learned, what happened. And it was a small town in which roots ran deep and history was closely personal, handed down to people who cared because they were concerned with the same houses, the same businesses, the same people.

In the small towns of America before World War II, the ribbon of family history was a constant in our lives. We were curious about what happened before we were born, and we listened. The country had not yet shrunk to one vast beckoning land, and our horizons were smaller. Our ancestors were buried in the local cemetery, and we expected to lie beside them. Ultimately we knew all there was to know about everybody with whom we came in contact.

The Library of Congress has four drawerfuls of reference works on the history of tuberculosis. The Adirondack Room in the Saranac Lake Library has many more. But the history of TB I am writing in this book was absorbed through the pores, was lived through and left scars on most of the people I loved. If I have made mistakes in the precise way that history unfolded, I don't think they change in any way the essence.

Tuberculosis took my mother from me during most of my youth, and even though I was nineteen when she died, I knew her scarcely at all. In the course of writing this book I came to know her. I was at first too young and then too removed to understand that the central fact of her life was tuberculosis. It altered her personality, her relationships, her world.

In digging into her past, I came little by little to see how this had happened. She began to emerge in my mind with new dimensions, and I took to wearing her little diamond wedding pendant, hung her black net dress beaded with jet that had lain so long neglected in my basement on a satin hanger in my closet. Halfway through the writing of the book, I brought her little watercolor of a Victorian lady from the dark corner where it hung downstairs and put it in a place of honor in the hall.

This then is not only a reprise of the greatest killer of the last century, but a discovery of a woman. How it would amuse her to see me trying on her dress in front of my mirror. I can imagine her laughing and saying again that she was glad I didn't inherit the Comstock thick ankles. And that really she had never liked that dress, the beads were always dropping off.

I'd like to tell her that I understand now, just a bit, what it was like to have tuberculosis before streptomycin.

𝓪 1

Everybody said my mother was pretty. I am not sure about that to this day, for the early sepia snapshots of her when she and my father were honeymooning at Key West have no resemblance to the mother I knew. I leaf through page after page of young women in long dresses and Gibson Girl hats, linking arms with men squinting into the sun beneath stiff boaters, and I am reduced to asking relatives which one she is.

"That one there," says my sister-in-law, who is older than I, pointing to a nearly buxom laughing young woman wearing a hat adorned with a bird of paradise.

I study the picture and have no choice but to believe her, for there is my father standing behind her and another couple I recognize. But there is nothing about her that looks familiar.

The mother I remember was very thin, somewhere around ninety-five pounds—thin, elegant and nervous. I see her seated at her dressing table leaning forward to dab some rouge on her cheeks, running a silver-backed comb through marcelled waves, rummaging impatiently through her drawer to find a necklace to fill in the neck of her yellow dress. I see her at our dining-room table opposite Father, pushing her food back and forth across the plate, selecting a bite here and there and conveying it listlessly to her mouth. In my mind she sits beside me in the back of our tall LaSalle with a running board, behind John, our Welsh chauffeur. She is wearing a squirrel coat and a close-fitting cloche, and her gloved fingers jump restlessly on the buffalo robe stretched across our knees.

There are only a few pictures in my mind of my mother when I was a little girl growing up in the twenties, for when my brother was six and I two, she was discovered to have tuberculosis and went to stay at a sanitarium in Saranac Lake, New York.* She had had a severe cold, and the cough hung on. It was a deep cough which alarmed my father, but she shrugged it off. She was what an earlier age called pleasingly plump and was dieting strenuously and soaking herself for long hours in a hot bath to melt away the pounds. The cough persisted, but the doctor in the small upstate New York town where we lived dismissed it as the result of too many parties and the severe winter.

And then one day, as she held on to the bedpost of the fourposter where she slept with my father, the blood welled up in her throat in a choking hemorrhage.

Doctors from Utica and then from New York City were

*Always referred to by the natives as simply Saranac, but not to be confused with another village in New York state located near Plattsburg and also called Saranac.

summoned. They came and went with serious faces, carrying their black bags. In a day or two Kathleen, our Irish second maid, packed my mother's dresses and her jewelry, her marabou-trimmed negligee and her set of Dickens, and she was borne away in the car to an Adirondack sanitarium to spend the next seven years.

In 1920, when my mother's car rolled up the steep hill to the Santanoni, an apartment hotel for health seekers (as it was advertised), Saranac Lake was a frigid village famous as a North American Lourdes for people seeking pulmonary cures. It was a one-industry town whose population was increasing daily. Every morning and evening train poured more desperate tubercular victims into the village, all of them hoping for a miraculous cure like that of Dr. Edward Livingston Trudeau.

Every new arrival knew the story of the bleak summer of 1875, when Trudeau came to nearby Paul Smith's, a sporting hostelry, to die of tuberculosis in the woods he had always loved. Saranac then was a hamlet consisting of a single schoolhouse, a sawmill and a small hotel for guides and lumbermen, almost fifty miles from the nearest railroad.

It was no easy trip from New York to the Adirondacks in those days. A train took Trudeau to Saratoga, where he stayed the night, pushing on to Whitehall the next day and then by boat through Lake Champlain to Plattsburg. After a two-day stopover to rest, he rode the little spur iron-ore road to Au Sable Forks, then traveled by carriage over a nearly impassable road forty-two miles to Paul Smith's. Small wonder that on his arrival Trudeau was so wasted with fever he had to be carried to his room. "Why, Doctor," said the man who climbed the stairs with him in his arms, "you don't weigh no more than a dried lambskin."

7

Consumption, as tuberculosis was called when Trudeau arrived at Paul Smith's, was almost invariably fatal. It was widely referred to as the White Plague, an oblique linking of its pale, life-draining characteristics to that of the scourge of civilization, the fourteenth-century Black Death. There was no recognized treatment for it, and Trudeau had, indeed, given up hope. Nevertheless the guides fixed him a bed of balsam boughs in a guide boat, laid his gun across the center seat and loaded him in to go hunting. Miraculously, slowly, day by day his health improved and he gained weight. When he was able to resume his medical practice, he attributed his recovery to the pure, cold mountain air and decided to settle in Saranac to found a sanitarium for other tuberculosis sufferers. The reputation of Saranac was established.

By the time my mother arrived in Saranac some forty years later, Dr. Trudeau had made the town into a world-famous cure center for consumptives. Nevertheless, though Koch had isolated the bacillus as far back as 1882, very little was actually still known about the disease. Belief in the miraculous effect of the climate amounted almost to a religion, and treatment consisted largely of building up the stamina of the patient. In spite of the glittering reputation of the Saranac sanitariums, cures were a sometime and random thing, relapses were frequent and death not unexpected.

People knew in the twenties what getting tuberculosis meant. It was a death knell, the end of a normal life and the beginning of months or years of enforced idleness, banishment and hopelessness. People with tuberculosis were isolated from the world, possibly as much for the sake of the general good as for hope of their own cure. Much was thought to depend on the early detection of the disease, and a hemorrhage meant the bacilli were well established. What must my mother have felt, a young married woman, sent to take the cure at Saranac, where the coffins were rolling out every night, two or three at a time, under cover of darkness from the spur of the New York Central Railroad?

"Sanitarium," Betty MacDonald, famous author of *The Egg and I,* was to say twenty years later when a doctor diagnosed her own case. "I knew what that meant. I had seen Margaret Sullavan in *Three Comrades* and I had read *The Magic Mountain.* Sanitariums were places in the Swiss Alps where people went to die. Not only that, but everyone I'd ever heard of who had had tuberculosis had died."

Plenty of them did. When Dr. Trudeau arrived at Saranac, tuberculosis was the leading cause of death in America. Fifty years later 88,000 Americans were still dying of it annually. Worse, no one really knew how the disease was contracted or how it could be cured. It struck mysteriously and killed indiscriminately. Many a car passed through Saranac in those days exceeding the speed limit as the driver pressed the accelerator to the floor and a clean handkerchief to his nose. The custom so irritated one old-time resident that one day he stood on the curb on Main Street and bawled after a disappearing car, "The tubernculars we got here probably came from your hometown!"

Like leprosy victims, the tuberculosis patient in my mother's day was often shunned. (Oddly enough, the bacilli for the two diseases are not unlike.) Many were the patients in Saranac whose families brought them thankfully to Trudeau Sanitarium, departed with relief and were never heard of again.

I was very young, and I do not remember much about Mother in that period, but I remember the fear. It dominated our lives. My father, Mother's hemorrhage still sickeningly etched in his mind, worried constantly that we children would also get the disease. Nobody at the time knew why tuberculosis struck some and not others, though it was well known to be infectious. Defenses against it were few and simple, and we observed them rigorously. A pitcher of milk sat on the table at every meal, and a sure way to win smiles all around was to help ourselves twice from it. Fresh air was likewise good: it was an amulet against illness, and our windows were flung wide each night even in subzero temperatures, so that we had to sleep in ski socks and sweaters. We were encouraged to eat heartily. Lack of appetite was one of the first alarming signs of consumption. Poundage was armor against infection.

Our household rearranged itself in my mother's absence. I acquired a nurse, whom I remember kindly for the way she did not much hurt when she brushed my hair and who, standing with me in the frigid bathroom mornings to dress, patiently helped me wrap my long johns neatly at the ankle. I don't think she believed much in tuberculosis. I never heard a word of it from her.

Downstairs, however, innumerable aunties and courtesy aunties filled the living room evenings, slipping their arms about my waist and murmuring endearments into my hair. "Poor darling baby," they said when they thought me out of earshot, as they sipped from cocktail glasses held in elegant, slim fingers. "Do you think she looks a tiny bit peaked, Ted? You must let me take her out and buy her a proper dress."

Plenty of rest was prescribed, and I was put to bed early, earlier by far than my friends. Each night my father personally heard my prayers, inserting by remote control a postscript on behalf of the family. ". . . and make Mother well and bring all the family together," I mumbled, down on my knees by the bed as he watched approvingly. I think he thought childish prayers went by a more direct line.

We went to visit Mother often. Saranac lies some hundred and fifty thickly forested miles north of Rome, where we lived. In the summer or on winter weekends when we children were not in school, my father drove us past the endless chain of clear lakes and the shadowy woods which lay between us and the Santanoni. My brother, by virtue of his years, sat beside Father on these trips. Alone in the back seat, I peered from the window at the woods, sniffing the pine and keeping a sharp eye out for the souvenir stores which clustered beside the road to sell deerskin gloves, bobcat-skin rugs and pine-stuffed pillows with "I Pine for You and Balsam" painted on them. When we stopped for gas we carefully avoided stations that kept, as many did in those days, a poor, scruffy baby bear chained to the pump awaiting the inevitable soda-pop handout from the customers.

Cramped from the long ride, we would stand at last in my mother's room at the Santanoni, awed and uneasy, each with a hand in Father's, well back from her bed against the wall. In the mental pictures I run of these moments, it is a big room and she is wearing her marabou-trimmed negligee and smiling at us. She has been sewing during the long hours of rest and holds up a little green crepe-de-Chine dress which has puff sleeves and smocking. I let loose of Father's hand and run to the bedside to take it while she holds it up to me, gauging the fit.

In the background I hear my father's voice. "Stand back," he says. "Don't get too close."

She gives me the dress, and I take my place again against the far wall, clutching it to my skinny chest, my hand once more in Father's. Later, on the way to the hotel where we are to spend the night, he regards the dress dubiously and says nothing.

"Wash your hands," he tells me when we are shown to our room.

Everywhere there are huge gaps I cannot fill in the years my mother spent in Saranac. I am sure she did not spend them all in bed, though that is where I mostly remember her. *The Journal of Outdoor Life,* a magazine for consumptives started by my mother's doctor, Lawrason Brown, shows pictures of tubercular patients bird-watching, picnicking, sleigh riding, even sledding. I do not think my mother went sledding, but there were certainly boat rides, drives and strolls on the beautiful mountain roads, and plenty of social gatherings at the Santanoni. The mountain air was the secret—one must get plenty of it. Hadn't it cured Dr. Trudeau? And, of course, as was well known, one winter was worth two summers in the Adirondacks, and one hour of driving worth two in the cure chairs, the wooden reclining chairs which lined the sleeping porches.

There is no continuity to what I remember, but any time I choose I can run the mental slides of my brother lying in a cure chair, wearing a fur hat with earflaps and attempting to turn the pages of the book he is reading without taking off his mittens. We are living part of the time in a house on Park Avenue in Saranac, and he is on the sleeping porch. The mercury in the thermometer is scarcely visible in the tube outside the screening. His cheeks are round and rosy, but the X-rays show a shadow on his lung. A trained nurse is living with us, and my father makes the journey alone through the woods every weekend to stay with us, in winter wearing the huge beaver coat which comes down to his heels that was a gift from his Canadian lumber connections. I scrub my hands so often they are raw, down glass after glass of milk and, though I am seven or eight, take afternoon naps.

Curled and cracked snapshots remain of me in a rowboat on nearby Lake Clear, my mother in the stern, her hair elaborately pompadoured, and my father and brother at the oars. I am smiling into the camera and wearing my boy's suit, of which I am terribly proud, but the smile is for the photographer. This is the summer that I begin to understand the fear. In my school they have discovered that my mother had tuberculosis and my brother a spot on his lung. I have been brought, dragging my feet and terrified, to be X-rayed, and, though the pictures are negative, now I, too, am worried.

"Do you think I have it yet?" I ask my brother, and he replies coldly, "I don't know. It is like water wearing away a stone."

The sight of my brother in a cure chair piled high with blankets makes it clear to me at last that it is possible that I could find myself in this same situation, confined to a sleeping porch with a book. What I took for granted in my mother I find frightening in my brother. I no longer have to be told to wash my hands. When my mother, peering into a beautiful red satin Valentine's box of candy we have brought her, selects one of my favorite kind and proffers it to me, I draw back as if burned.

It is like water wearing away a stone. My brother has told me. I know the rules.

In my hearing my mother never spoke of her life in Saranac. I piece it together from the unguarded comments of my aunts, from rare confidences from my lonely father. My brother is silent on the subject. "There are some things," he says, "I do not like to think about." He recovered completely within two years, but those years are blacked out, sealed off like the scar on his lung. When my mother came home, still a semi-invalid, I was sent to summer camp and from there to boarding school. And so it was not until I was grown and the fear had been laid to rest forever that I came to wonder how it was to be a young woman in Saranac in the early twenties, a young woman who had left her family behind for the layered society of the country's most famous tuberculosis cure center.

In June of 1976 in Saranac I stood at the bottom of the hill to look once more up at the Santanoni. It had been gutted by fire and stood, deserted but still proud, like a *grande dame* down on her luck, its windows blackened with smoke and its top two stories gone. I walked up the drive in search of a piece of my mother's life and found the new owner puttying the broken windows.

He had been a small boy who came frequently to the back kitchen door for a pastry treat in the twenties, and he remembered vividly the Santanoni in its full flower. It was very grand, he told me, shaking his head. Such a kitchen! Every day his father sold the chef fresh fish caught in the lake. Opening onto the lobby had been one of the first hydraulic elevators in the country, and the patients who rode it were most elegantly dressed. They were forever having cocktail parties and smoking, like my mother, from those long, slim cigarette holders which appear in John Held, Jr., drawings. Those on the top floors brought their own private nurses.

The list of tuberculars he remembered could have been cribbed from an international *Who's Who*. He seemed to find the names in odd corners of his mind, the decades of their Saranac sojourn melding into one timeless parade: Stella Adler, daughter of the great Jacob Adler of the Yiddish theatre; Hope Lange, the movie and television actress; Christy Mathewson, the baseball player; Rosalind Russell's adopted daughter; the wife of the chef of the New York Ritz, Louis Diat, my mother's particular friend; Manuel Quezon, the president of the Philippines, who brought his retinue and established a government in absentia at the nearby Hotel Saranac; Dean Acheson's daughter, Mrs. William Bundy.

In the office of the *Adirondack Enterprise* next day, searching through the files, I found the account of the fire and the obituary of the Santanoni.

It had been designed by William Scopes, who took a correspondence course in architecture while lying in a Trudeau bed and later became a well-known architect. Its quartered-oak floors became legendary after it opened in 1914. Its elevator was a first. From the moment it was completed, a long list of patients sought apartments there. It boasted the latest in cure accommodations, with one and sometimes two sleeping porches for every room and beds on wheels that could be rolled out for the patient to enjoy the air. Two regular nurses were in constant attendance, and the doctors who called daily were the aristocracy of the profession: Lawrason Brown, who had succeeded Trudeau at the sanitarium; Francis Trudeau, senior and junior; Hugh Kinghorn; J. N. Hayes; J. Woods Price.

"Dr. Brown," I hear my mother saying, "is an important man in Saranac."

Very expensive, the Santanoni, says the new owner, shaking his head. Think of the labor just to shovel that driveway from the street. And the meals they used to have. Always three and four courses. And the people who met in the cure chairs lined up on the sleeping porches, each with its hot stone flask at the feet in winter. One such new friendship resulted in the marriage of June Serrelas of the Don Q rum fortune to a fellow patient. The red carpet ran all the way from St. Bernard's Church at the end of the block to the Hotel Saranac, where the reception was held; and for the occasion the Serrelas family presented the church with a new $10,000 organ for the playing of the wedding march.

And did most of the patients get well? I asked him. But he didn't know. It was a long time ago, and few remember. Many came and stayed awhile and went back where they came from too soon. Tuberculosis was a disease particularly prone to remission and then recurrence. They came and went. Legs Diamond's brother had a house just down the block, and so did Harry Houdini's brother. Mrs. Francis Trudeau, daughter-in-law of the founder of Trudeau Sanitarium, says she played bridge regularly in 1914 with Dutch Queen Wilhelmina, the head of the Bank of France, whose name escapes her, and a curator from Buckingham Palace. In the winter of 1887 Robert Louis Stevenson spent months in a rambling cottage nearby, believing himself to be tubercular, though there is doubt about that now.

Walk along Main Street in Saranac today and it is hard to imagine such people rubbing elbows here. A town of just over 6,000, with a winter temperature that hovers for days at ten below zero, Saranac is an ordinary town from which history has moved on. It has the depressed look of many other upstate cities whose factories have been shut down.

The air is still cold, crisp and clean, the same sharp mountain air that drew train after train of "lungers" here early in the century. But now there are streptomycin and isoniazid, rifampin and ethambutol, and a discovery of a tubercular lesion on the lung means nothing more inconvenient than a year or more's course of drugs while the patient scarcely interrupts his life stride. As a death threat, tuberculosis is through, except perhaps in parts of the Third World. Only the old-timers in Saranac remember when things were different.

"Dr. Brown says I am improving," writes my mother to my father somewhere in the early twenties. "I am forcing myself to eat and have put on five pounds. If only he would let me come home soon."

2 ❧

My mother was inclined to shyness up until the time of her marriage, which took place on Christmas Eve early in the second decade of the century. It was a wedding of some interest, partly because my father's people were locally fashionable, and partly because he had resisted the idea of marriage until he was thirty-seven. When he went to call on his father to tell him of his engagement, the old gentleman, a dignified man who had inherited a wholesale lumber business, gazed at him over the top of his *New York Herald Tribune* and remarked, "Well, you're old enough."

My mother was almost ten years my father's junior, and he took her into what was then referred to as an older set. They were monied, easygoing, pleasure-loving people who had either inherited or made comfortable fortunes in an era when the income tax was not troublesome. They spent much of the winter in Palm Beach or Key West or Nassau, and their homes were more than comfortable, largely close together on North George Street, which was where the gentry in Rome, New York, lived. It was they who organized the country club, led the charity balls over the old Strand Theatre, gave the most amusing parties. The men were mill owners who ran their business so successfully that the burgeoning unions could not organize their employees, and the *Wolverine* and the *Commodore Vanderbilt,* hurtling west on the tracks to Chicago, shrieked to a special hissing stop in Rome at their request.

This is not to say that they took themselves seriously. It was like belonging to the best fraternity. You went to an Ivy League college, you married the prettiest girl, things went right all the way and, in addition, you could come home for lunch.

"Ah, they were the ones we watched," sighed a woman who peered through the curtains at it all as a younger sister. "They were so gay."

My mother, like the rest of the women, was completely uneducated by today's standards. Except for a few bluestockings, women in her day did not go to college. She was bookish, but fortunately she was also pretty and witty. She married my father, sat on the front porch of the country club as the bolder of her contemporaries took up golf, embroidered tea towels and saw that the cook put proper meals before us.

They drove the first motor cars under the arched elms of North George Street, bought saddle horses, gave each other elaborate and expensive surprise presents. They went fishing together in the Adirondacks, sitting for long hours in the sun on crystal lakes, the men wearing straw boaters and old khakis from Abercrombie and the women huge hats to shade their faces. The richer among them followed the seasons around the world on cruises during which they met amusing people who later came to visit them.

Their homes were full of servants and of children who wore sailor suits and hand-smocked dresses with white Buster Brown shoes. The demands of domesticity were sweet but not highly time-consuming.

A year after my parents were married, my brother was born. He, too, wore a sailor suit and posed for a picture sitting in a huge wicker peacock chair holding a puppy in his lap, his fat ankles encased in high shoes. It was tacitly understood that he would go to Andover and Yale as his father had.

My parents moved to a bigger house on Maple Street, and down at the lumberyard where my father was vice president, things went smoothly. The New York Central cars rolled often over railroad ties purchased in Canada and sold by my father's mill. Twice a month he would board the *Empire State*, the crack train between New York and Chicago, and call on railroad officials and renew old acquaintances at the Yale Club in New York City. He would return without fail on Friday night on the *Commodore Vanderbilt* in time for dinner.

The summers in Rome were golden, and the winters, from October through March, were frigid and snowbound. Milk delivery was by a wagon with runners, and the city snowplows moved constantly through the streets, building drift piles at the side of the thoroughfares twice as high as a man's head. Down at the Busy Corner, the junction of James and Dominick streets, traffic moved as usual under these conditions. The snow was packed down smoothly on the streets, and the coal furnaces kept the houses toasty enough to allow bare arms at the formal Saturday-night parties my mother's crowd hosted in rotation.

It was a secure and affluent world in which my mother dwelt. The telephone, whose receiver hung by a hook on the side, rang constantly, and if you couldn't reach your friends, Operator usually knew where they had gone. There were afternoon excursions to purchase delicacies for the table and even possibly a new hat. My brother was in Miss McFarland's nursery school, and a cook reigned in the kitchen.

In the front parlor, standing before the long pier-glass mirror which her mother had given her when she was married, my mother turned sidewise to inspect her figure and admire the dresses she bought in New York. Was her waist as slim as before the birth of the baby? Would the Gibson Girl shirtwaist be more becoming if she dropped a pound or two? She took to dieting, sipping hot lemonade and spending hours in a hot tub reading Dickens while she tried to sweat the pounds off.

Every other Friday night she met the *Commodore Vanderbilt* thundering up the valley from New York en route to Chicago, picking her way through the snowy walks in winter to the railroad depot without overshoes, her gray squirrel coat hanging open so that one could see her thin pink chiffon blouse. What was life if one must be sensible all the time? One could catch a cold sitting home listening to the radio. The stationmaster shook his head when she went by, but the long, haunting whistle of the *Commodore* was already signaling a stop, and she picked up her skirts and scampered up the marble stairs to the platform for westbound trains, to fall into my father's arms as the conductor opened the door.

Then she was pregnant again. They had talked of two children, sometime in the future perhaps. But already their son was four years old, and Dr. Black—who had started his practice when you could still be an internist, gynecologist and surgeon all in one—was sure she was pregnant. She felt like an animal in a trap, but, little by little, she became resigned. And just as the sun was rising one February morning, in the brand-new city hospital where more and more women were going to have their children, she presented my father with a daughter.

For a girl there were smocked dresses to make and small sunbonnets to be bought. I was named after her, and, though a sore disappointment to my brother because I couldn't play ball right away, I took my place in the household. Mother and Father left us with a nurse and went off to Key West, where they had honeymooned and where Dr. Black hoped she would shake the last cold, which seemed to hang on.

When they came back she was still coughing and seemed to have been unable to eat much of the hotel food. It was not very good, she said. But it was summer by now, and there were picnics at Big Brook and long afternoons at the country club sitting on the porch and waiting for the men to finish their golf. And at Christmas she had a red velvet dress for the charity ball, and afterward she and all her friends walked through the arcade to the Stanwix Hotel for a midnight supper. So there wasn't time to think about a cold that hung on.

The frequent shopping trips to New York seemed to exhaust her more and more, and Dr. Black pulled a long face and said she really must take care of her cold. But I was toddling about underfoot and needed white shoes, and there was a plan to move the club farther out into the country near an artificial lake. My mother shrugged off the cold and said that she was all right, just tired.

But the cough got deeper and looser and seemed to shake her entire frame with its spasms. She was picking at her food, and occasionally she would wake in the night beside my father in the big bed, drenched with sweat.

One morning, after he had gone to work, she was peering into her closet deciding on a dress when a particularly bad fit of coughing racked her. She clung to the bedpost, her eyes widening, feeling things rearranging themselves inside her. Seconds later she was staring, stunned, at a thick red pool of her own blood settling into the sun-washed colors of the Oriental rug.

3 ❀

In those days the specter of tuberculosis was as terrifying as cancer is today. Every third person between the ages of fifteen and sixty in the country—or about one in ten—died of TB. It was widely known to kill and, prior to their death, to disable its victims and reduce them to a state of helplessness. It was a wasting disease that was also highly contagious, which meant that sufferers were usually ostracized.

It is thus not hard to imagine what my mother was thinking as she clung to the bedpost in her thin negligee, staring at the blood at her feet.

In the bleak horror of this prospect, there was one light of hope. Saranac Lake was the Switzerland of America, and if you lived east of the Mississippi River, you went there whether or not you could afford it, carried on a stretcher if necessary, for it was the only chance. The most brilliant doctors in the country were practicing there, specialists from New York and Montreal who had followed Trudeau to his sanitarium—usually men who, like him, had suffered from the disease personally, come to Saranac and stayed on to practice because this was the acknowledged center for TB work.

There was never any question that my mother would go to Saranac. It was only a matter of arranging.

Gazing down at her, lying white and exhausted on the bed, my father turned away to set the wheels in motion.

Only the best would do, he vowed. That was paramount. Naturally he would not expect Dr. Trudeau to take care of her himself, but the best after him. Who was Lawrason Brown, whose name everyone was murmuring? The man who had succeeded Trudeau at the head of the Institute? Did everyone have confidence in him? A Hopkins man whom Osler had spoken highly of? It began to sound possible. And it was good to know that he had suffered from TB himself. Then he would know how it felt to find the blood gushing from your mouth when you were only trying to select a gown from your closet. He was the man.

From the big bed, my mother's hand fluttered and attached itself to his sleeve.

"How long?" she whispered, gazing up at him from the pillow, so pale that only her blond hair, spread wide, delineated her features. "How long will I have to stay?"

He did not know. It was not a point anyone had seen fit to mention. He shook his head gently, squeezing her hand, and she shut her eyes.

Two days later they loaded her into the Studebaker and

drove cautiously over the wooded back roads to begin her indefinite stay at what the *Adirondack Enterprise* called the City of the Sick.

When my father turned the nose of the blue Studebaker off the road from Tupper Lake onto Main Street in Saranac, the village was at the height of its fame. Almost one in three persons living in Saranac had consumption, as it was then called. The remaining two were engaged in one way or another in taking care of the sick, or so it was said.

It didn't look like the answer to Switzerland to my mother. It looked like the end of a road that she had not known she was traveling, an undistinguished village with a narrow, branched main street and the buildings crowding the sidewalk. She peered from the car window, blinking back the tears, and watched as a drugstore or two, a modest hotel, a barbershop with a huge bowl of goldfish in the window passed in succession and were gone. The people in the street seemed preoccupied and roughly dressed. Rome was no metropolis, but by comparison this was chilly, bleak and alien. As they rounded the corner into Church Street, she pulled her coat close.

An attractive house on the corner, she thought, and read the sign as my father shifted gears—Dr. Edward Trudeau. So this was the home of the great man. Two or three more well-kept-up houses and then the sanitarium, her sanitarium, her home for a period which nobody so far had been willing to estimate.

Up a high, high hill, the Studebaker straining in second gear, and into the courtyard in front of a handsome Tudor-like building with mullioned bay windows flanked by tall hemlocks. She gripped the door handle and stepped from the car as my father opened the door. She was determined to walk, though her knees felt uncertain. She stood quietly for a moment, looking at the big door, waiting for the strength to return and stiffen her bones. She turned to look for my father and for the first time saw the mountains, blue-hazed and beautiful, on the near horizon.

"It's pretty here, Bess," my father said, taking her hand. "You'll be happy here."

She nodded and burst into tears.

My mother did not know or care on the late fall day when she arrived at the Santanoni Apartment House for Health Seekers, but the Saranac Lake of which she had just caught a glimpse was as lusty, monied and wide open as any frontier town. It encompassed a glittering international set, some of the world's most famous doctors, a smattering of high-echelon underworld and a large representation from the New York stage and Hollywood screen. Many important people sought healing in Saranac, but many, too, for whom $15 a week board and room at a cottage sanitarium was a constant worry. Forced to give up their jobs, hundreds lived here on the charity of relatives or, out in the wards of Ray Brook sanitarium, on the charity of the state. The wards of Ray Brook were full of desperately ill tuberculars, once self-sufficient, who had abandoned themselves to institutional care.

The village to which my mother had come was already bursting at the seams, but every day two trains brought more of the sick. Many arrived on stretchers and had to be lifted out through the windows to waiting ambulances. Hundreds more came lying on cots in the baggage car, and not a few returned that same night, rolled in shrouds, in the same car.

The population of Saranac was as changing as the sands of the beach; this was the place of hope, but some had delayed too long.

From the brown-shingled affluence of Park Avenue where the swells lived, to the lowliest two-bed roominghouse calling itself a "san," the entire social structure of Saranac geared itself to TB. Nine druggists dispensed fever thermometers, sputum cups and stone hot-water bottles known as pigs to keep the feet of patients warm in the long outdoor nights. Taxicabs without number idled at every corner of Broadway and Main, awaiting the crooked finger of the ambulatory patient on exercise permission. Every night the Pontiac Theatre played to a full house with a waiting line. ("The theatre beautiful with a $12,000 orchestral organ, perfect ventilation and the largest screen in Central New York.")

For some, however, the main streets of Saranac were as remote as the steppes of Siberia. Their world was bounded by the walls of their rooms. Enough of them eventually died to keep three undertakers busy preparing the remains for shipment back to where they came from.

It was a world center, but it was still a small village.

Down at C. J. Carey's or T. F. Finnigan's, a suit with two pairs of pants cost $50—unless you were one of the veterans the government was subsidizing and then it was double. The telephone system fed through operators who still knew nearly all the people in town and their one- to three-digit telephone numbers. A lot of bigwigs had come to the village, and in the evening, when you walked the streets, you could look through the windows and see them tucked in bed reading. If you weren't going to the movies, the big amusement was to go down to watch the train come in and take a look at the latest arrivals straggling in a line two blocks from the depot to the

St. Regis Hotel, whose stationery announced that it did not receive tubercular guests but which housed many who did not cough too publicly.

"What a town it was," says Tony Anderson, who has been Mayor of Saranac Lake a half-dozen times. "The whole village was a san. It was like the Klondike, a money town."

Tony ought to know. Born with the century, he contracted TB, came to Saranac and stayed on like so many when he got well.

There was money, all right. Up on millionaires' row on Park Avenue, things were nice, if rustic. Ancient elms arched over the street, shading benches provided for convalescents who found themselves tiring partway through their walk. Mailboxes discreetly displayed famous names: P. J. Lorillard of tobacco fame, whose son had TB; Walter Cluett, whose shirts dressed gentlemen of fashion and whose wife had it; Christy Mathewson, when he moved from the Santanoni.

They came and they went. The houses changed hands according to the health of their occupants, and the narrow streets of the village were clogged with Cords, Duesenbergs, Pierce Arrows and Packards with the spare tires in the running-board well.

Some of the money was the reward of industrial success, and some came from the wrong side of the law. The Riverside Inn, on pretty little Lake Flower near the center of the town, rented an entire floor to the wife of Eddie Diamond, Legs Diamond's brother, who was taking the cure. There were seven stills in town and a thriving bootleg business. Saranac imported plenty of liquor from Montreal and manufactured a lot more. Every drugstore sold booze packaged in nursing bottles, and the dry-cleaning establishment prospered because regular customers paid large fees to receive their suits back cleaned and pressed with a pint tucked in the pocket. Police Chief James Couglin employed seven patrolmen, but underworld connections were powerful and well established and did not hesitate to provide a pair of cement shoes for the nosy. Saranac in the twenties was a hard-drinking, two-fisted town with a to-hell-with-tomorrow psyche.

The favorite watering hole of what the village called the lungers was the Berkeley Hotel on Main Street, where Tom Ward, who owned it, founded the Saranac Club especially for them. Patients taking the cure loved to drop in and refresh themselves while they watched the world go by under the windows—and most of the world suffering from TB actually did go by, as well as the doctors, who were the deities, the arbiters of fate. Most lived around the corner on Church Street, as close together after they turned out the lights as they were in their labors, all clustered close to Dr. Edward Trudeau's corner residence.

Down the street, katty-corner from the little Episcopal Church of St. Luke the Beloved Physician and directly across from Dr. Trudeau, dwelt Dr. Brown. Each morning he left his yellow house early to climb the steep hill to the Santanoni to see my mother.

4

Saranac Lake—host to some of the underworld notorious and yet a place where a lost umbrella nearly always found its way back to its owner—was at first only a fleeting and distant impression to my mother. Dr. Brown—a gentle, nervous man with a mustache, dark hair parted in the middle and obviously painful feet—had arrived on her first day and decreed absolute bed rest, forbidding her to put so much as a foot outside the bedclothes. Worst of all, he had surveyed the bedside table with its towering pile of books overshadowing the fever thermometer in its neat jar and suggested curtailed reading laced with long periods of simply lying with closed eyes. He listened to her chest, looked down at her gravely as if she were an interesting microscopic specimen and departed in a flurry of respectful nurses.

At first she wept, thinking of the two children at home, the parties going on without her, the maples turning silver and red outside the door of her new home. But they warned her against tears, pointing out that an infant crying doubles his metabolic rate, a bad thing for a consumptive. The days stretched unending, each exactly like its predecessor, punctuated only by trays, the proffered thermometer and Dr. Brown's visits. She lay watching the headlights of the cars on Church Street reflected on the ceiling of her room while the gathering dusk outside turned the mountains purple. She wondered if she would die, die by inches, lying in this bed. When she turned to the wall, strange sounds rattled inside her, gurglings that frightened her. Fluid in the lungs, said the nurses, patting the covers over her shoulder reassuringly.

It was the standard treatment in the 1920s—absolute bed rest for a minimum of six weeks which could stretch into months if the fever persisted. Even raising your arms was forbidden, and a deep breath was not allowed because the lesion in the lungs might be stretched and pour out its poisons. The body's defenses must be given every chance to work against the invading germs. The pace must be slowed to near hibernation while the struggle went on unseen within the patient.

Fear kept the patients lying as they were told. For it was well known that many died. They could point all they wanted to the ones who got well, but it was not hard to see the gaps in the ranks every day. At Trudeau Institute the patients took their own morning head count daily when their beds were rolled onto the porches. Every night the wheels of the ice wagon rattled over the street bringing chunks of ice for the chest of some patient suffering a final and fatal hemorrhage. Sometimes it was a special friend who had slipped away on a sea of red blood, leaving an empty bed.

Accordingly, Mother, a rebel accustomed to flouting authority, lay quiescent and obediently inert for two months, drifting in a world regulated by the rise and fall of the mercury in her fever thermometer. Every afternoon at four the silver in the little stick began its steady climb up the scale to one hundred plus. A hundred meant bed rest. For the future, Dr. Brown said, they would see. For now she must try to be patient.

They taught her to cough in the morning to raise a sputum sample for the Gafne test of germ count, and thereafter to eschew coughing at all costs. "A man who coughs hard all day does as much work as a man who climbs a mountain," said Dr. Brown. Every erg of energy was needed to fight the disease. They brought her ice, pieces of slippery elm, sips of cold milk to stop the coughs before they escaped from her lungs.

She lay as quiet as her muscles and her thoughts would allow, imagining the crysanthemums blooming in the back garden and the new nurse my father had found for us children. After a while she despaired, but they were used to that, too, and did their best to cheer her, pointing out that thousands had healed and that she, too, in all probability, would. She thought bitterly of Camille and of Elizabeth Barrett Browning and how unlike that world of reclining chaise longues, camellias and fans consumption truly was. When she opened her eyes, they brought her another glass of milk, urging her to drink up, she must gain weight.

Dr. Brown came and went with regularity, but beyond studying the fever chart and listening to her chest, he said little. The strange gurgling noises in her chest continued, and the days slipped by, one exactly like the other. And still he would not let her stir. She began to wish she were dead. She thought briefly of stepping into thin air off her little balcony, for of what use was it to be young and alive if one is unable to move about?

It was banishment, solitary confinement too cruel to imagine.

Of this she said little to my father. At the end of her first two weeks he sat again in the chair by the bed, smoking endless cigarettes, his face thin and taut under his fading tan.

"Are you all right, Bess?" he asked her anxiously, and she gave him the ghost of a smile.

He spent the rest of the day telling her reassuring things he had invented.

The rigid regimen was standard in Saranac, and some of the famous doctors were even more strict. Dr. H. M. Kinghorn was generally thought to be the most severe. His patients, the story went, were allowed to crook a finger on one hand after a year and one on the other hand the second. The in-joke in Saranac in the twenties was that one of Dr. Kinghorn's patients tried to buy a new suit at T. F. Finnigan's and, when he was recognized as a Kinghorn patient, was directed instead to the pajama counter. It is quite possible, they say today in Saranac Lake, that some of Dr. Kinghorn's patients are still tucked away in rooms about the town.

Unlike cancer and other fatal diseases involving pain and gradual undermining of the body's strength, the trauma of tuberculosis fell most strongly on the mind. The forced inactivity allowed plenty of time for thinking and worrying, and there was plenty of reason to worry. Tuberculosis was a disease which shut off your working life and separated you from your family, who might or might not keep your memory green during the long years of cure. Add to this the very natural worry over death and the fact that the poisons of the lung cavities were thought to attack the nervous system, making it less reliable, and it is no wonder the beds of Saranac were filled with people undergoing severe emotional crises as they tried to adjust to their situation.

In an era that had yet to discover psychology for the masses, great stress was laid by the doctors on cheerfulness under difficulties. In some cases, weeks in bed turned into months and even years, and the learned articles of the day repeatedly insisted that the body's defenses could be better marshaled to overcome the bacilli if the mind of the unwilling host maintained a positive outlook. Dr. Walter H. James, president of Trudeau in 1924, in a speech pleading for financial support of the sanitarium, remarked:

"This disease consists of a struggle, an almost equal battle, between the invading germs and a man's body and extending over many months or even years. The tuberculosis bacilli feed less willingly and eagerly on cheerful, happy than upon depressed and gloomy tissues."

My mother, for some time, offered the germs depressed and gloomy tissue to feed on.

"Dr. Brown will not yet say when I can leave the bed," read the letter she dictated to the nurse. "I do nothing all day but lie here staring at the mountains and I wish they would rearrange them a bit."

I would not be surprised if she had wanted to say that she thought she would die, but the nurse would never have approved.

Rest, food and fresh air—these were all there were to

combat the disease which John Bunyan called "the Captain of All the Men of Death." Hope of cure was based on the circumstantial evidence of Dr. Trudeau's miraculous recovery at Paul Smith's and on his famous experiment in 1885 with rabbits.

The rabbits had been divided into three lots of five. The first lot was inoculated with pure tuberculosis cultures, let loose on a small island in front of Dr. Trudeau's camp at Paul Smith's, supplied with plenty of food that rabbits fancy and allowed to pursue their own business in the fresh air and sunshine.

The second lot was also inoculated with tuberculosis, but these poor creatures were put in a dark, damp place, confined in a box with bad air and very little food.

The third lot shared the second's unhappy conditions, but had not been inoculated.

In lot one, all but one rabbit survived. In lot two, four died within three months with evidence of tuberculosis. The third lot of rabbits emerged from the test emaciated, but with no signs of the disease.

The news was scarcely out when the sound of hammer and saw resounded through the village. As far as Saranac could see, the healthful mountain air of Saranac had been endorsed. Before long scarcely a home could be found in town without its bulging sleeping-porch addition, built in the name of health and—not really as an afterthought—profit.

5

The medical men of the twenties placed their faith in the
Saranac climate, which they thought of as God-given armor
against the ravages of the tuberculosis bacilli. Ironically, the
worst aspects of the climate were the very ones which most
recommended themselves to the doctors.

"The Adirondack summer season is shorter than in any
other portion of the United States, being approximately 110
days between spring and fall frosts," wrote Dr. Charles C.
Trembley, one of the famous Saranac names of the day in an
article titled "Distinctive Factors Which Bear on Saranac
Lake As a Health Center." "The cold of winter, though
registering a very low point on the thermometer, is not

penetrating but affords a brisk tonicity to both body and appetite."

The tonicity of the climate, if there is such a thing, was not immediately apparent to everyone. Robert Louis Stevenson, who had come to Saranac in 1887 to take the cure in a house not far from the railroad track, complained that the weather was "bleak, blackguard and beggarly."

"You should see the cows butt against the walls in the early morning while they feed," he wrote in a letter to Henry James. "You should also see our back log when the thermometer goes (as it does go) away away below zero til it can be seen no more by the eye of man—not the thermometer which is still perfectly visible, but the mercury—which curls up into the bulb like a hibernating bear."

The boy who did the chores, he went on to complain, had two answers to questions on the weather—cold or lovely, which meant raining. It rained often, when it wasn't snowing—an average annual rainfall of thirty-four inches, which, the Saranac Lake Chamber of Commerce pointed out, purged the atmosphere of dusts and harmful bacteria. And above all, of course, there were those wide temperature swings, considered highly healthful.

The snows came—still come—in October and didn't disappear until May, and the only possible garb to be worn on the streets was earmuffs, galoshes and a fur coat with special windguards sewed into the sleeves. The doctors all drove Franklin motor cars which were air-cooled and thus proof against the terrible cold which froze the ordinary cars. All cars had to navigate not on plowed roads but on thoroughfares in which successive snowfalls had been simply packed down by the horse-drawn plows into a gigantic flat pathway between huge snowbanks. The pavements emerged in May some twelve inches or so below their winter level.

The Switzerland of America had two seasons, the wags said—July and winter.

The natives—having been born to it and profiting from brisk sales of articles useful for coping with the cold—trudged stolidly through the snow, but the patients, forced to spend eight hours outdoors whatever their former inclinations, cursed the thermometer. Local stores did an enormous business in long johns, sportsmen's wool socks for bed, mittens, fur hats with earflaps and special Klondike blankets for wrapping one's self like a mummy while taking the cure. The doctors even instructed their patients in the approved way of wrapping for maximum warmth and assured them that, if they were properly protected, the cold could only hasten their recovery. Dr. Edward Trudeau's statue outside the Institute depicts him wrapped in a blanket in a cure chair, but the folds are artistically draped, not really according to the approved diagram in the patient's handbooks.

The private sanitariums, which took their cue from Trudeau and whose patients were usually cared for by members of the Trudeau staff in their private-practice hours, all provided places where their clients could spend eight hours in the killing, bitter cold. Those patients who did not have the money to stay at a sanitarium equipped with porches passed their days in bed with the windows constantly opened wide, closing them only when visitors came or sometimes when they were celebrating holidays. Neighboring stores did a brisk business in window tents which enabled patients to sleep with their heads sticking out the windows on a light platform covered with netting and a canvas top. Dr. Brown, in his handbook for patients, refers to these as a possible substitute for sleeping on a porch, though he does remark, "What room suffices him who knows a porch?"

At Trudeau, at Ray Brook, at the private sanitariums

within the village, the patients lay like recumbent audiences in their cure chairs on the porches, watching winter's frosty performance unfold. At Ray Brook, in the early days, it was actually total immersion, for the beds were all in tents. The belief that the cold was salubrious was so ingrained that occasionally an over-enthusiastic disciple would open his fur coat and sweater to bare his chest to the zero weather.

Nowhere is it written that the doctors practiced what they preached. "Do you know how wide my husband opened the window in our bedroom?" whispers pretty Mrs. Kinghorn, the eminent doctor's widow. "This wide," holding her thumb and forefinger less than an inch apart.

But during the day the famous doctors spoke so movingly of the benefits of cold, pure mountain air that there were those who, unable to afford the open-air accommodations, did the next best thing they could by creeping to the door often and throwing it wide to inhale fresh draughts of the healing currents.

"Sleeping out horrifies the spoiled children of civilization," wrote a patient of the Adirondack Cottage Sanitarium (as Trudeau was called in 1906), "but, once adopted, it appeals to every primal human instinct."

"Properly clad persons can be quite comfortable sitting outdoors even at twenty or thirty below," said Dr. Brown.

To my mother, the cold was nothing particularly new, a mere grace note to a climate with which she had long been familiar. In her home in the Mohawk Valley the cold had always been a fact of life which she understood. True, she had never before had to lie outdoors in it for eight hours, her breath freezing as it left her lips and her hands too cold to hold her book except through the folds of the blanket. But most of it she had experienced before, and if she fretted, it was not because of the cold. What bothered her was the third tenet of Dr. Brown's cure program, which he had put aptly for her into a small three-line sing-song:

> Eat once for yourself,
> Eat once for the germs
> Eat once to gain weight.

My mother had no more appetite than a molting canary and eating once was more than she could do. She could not remember when she had been hungry, when the smell of cooking food had not made her want to turn away. For months, untempted by the choicest out-of-season foods, the most inspired cooking, she had been pushing the food about her plate, rearranging it, redistributing it so that it looked tasted. And now what small appetite she had mustered before was diminished by the fever, and she longed to drop the bits of fresh fish, lamb chops, *petit fours* they brought her into the wastebasket, under the pillow, anywhere where she would not have to deal with them and they would not be noticed.

Yet to eat was the third commandment, part of the bargain which she must honor in order to leave this place or even the bed. It governed her life and the life of the others like her who were lying in beds from Hemorrhage Hill to the Riverside Inn. The nurses would never let her forget it, hovering nearby as she picked at her plate, pleading for her to take just one more morsel, force one tiny bite more. Dr. Brown hoped she would put on ten pounds—she who had feared to add an inch to her fashionably tiny waist. She was required to stuff herself like a Thanksgiving turkey, and it made her virtually sick.

"Eat up," urged the white-capped nurses. "We'll be weighing you soon," and they handed her the eternal eggnog or cup of steaming cocoa. "Eat up and you will be able to get out of bed."

"How could I possibly have any appetite lying here?" complained my mother to my father.

But it was the rule. Six glasses of milk daily, six raw eggs. Cream soups, Hollandaise, chocolate cake with icing.

"I can't do it," she told my father, who seemed to be smoking more and losing weight. "It disgusts me. And I won't fit into my clothes."

Neither of them mentioned the thought that was uppermost in both their minds. If she did not do as they said, she would have no use for the clothes.

The nurses, who had unpacked the rows of slim chiffon evening gowns, the angora dresses and shirtwaists which fitted so closely, did not tell my mother all they knew. They had seen the rows of little pointed shoes in the closet, the pretty walking skirts made to fit my mother's tiny waist, and they held their peace.

Nevertheless they were well aware that all over town patients had come, like her, for the cure and, urged by their doctors, finally accumulated enough weight to attain a figure which could only be called gross. There were patients who, after several months of stuffing themselves like Strasbourg geese, could no longer fit into even their shoes. "Eat well, it's weighing day," was the watchword out at Trudeau, and many of the consumptives, tired of swallowing three and four glasses of water to coax the scales to weight heavier, ate till they vomited.

"The more fat that can be absorbed unconsciously, the better," admonished a booklet entitled *How to Get Well,* published in Saranac in 1906. "A good cook," says the anonymous author, a recuperating patient, "can use a lot of oil in cooking." Apparently many did, then and later, though the practice of dosing with cod-liver oil was abandoned before the turn of the century. Irving Altman, normally a slight, wiry man, weighed 184 when he finished his cure. Today he still runs Saranac's leading dress shop on Broadway, and he might tip the scale at 140. Mrs. Morris Dworski, who worked in the chemical lab at Will Rogers Hospital for tuberculars, ballooned from her usual weight in the 120's to 185 at the end of her regimen.

It was a popular saying that you couldn't tell the ambulatory patients from their visiting relatives except that the ones who looked most healthy were likely to be the consumptives.

6 ✤

My mother's suite at the Santanoni—bedroom, living room, porch and private bath—seemed like a prison to her, but to hundreds of others lying in cure chairs in the early twenties at Saranac it would have looked like an apartment in heaven.

It is hard to imagine now what a difference it made in the twenties to have enough money when you were sick. Being too sick to work was like being caught on a double-barbed fishhook—as you lay helpless, the money dwindled away and the future became a dark tunnel through which you drifted toward bankruptcy, with absolutely no guarantee of ever regaining your health. Even the simplest sanitarium with two beds in a room cost between $7 and $15 a week exclusive of doctors' bills—a seemingly insignificant sum by today's standards, but if you are sick and Blue Cross has not yet been invented, it is a sum that is hard to come by. My mother was suffering undeniable trauma, but she was experiencing it surrounded by every comfort my father could buy for her.

In Ray Brook, the huge compound of a sanitarium on the road to Lake Placid which the State of New York maintained for indigent patients, the trains rolled in daily on a special spur of the New York Central to unload dozens of late-diagnosed consumptives caught in this double-pronged nightmare. They were bedded in wards to await the kind of decisions on their future usually suffered only by privates in the army. Each bed patient cost the state money, and the knife was the quick way, so operations usually reserved for last-ditch measures were said to be performed early on in Ray Brook. The patients did not enjoy cure options available nearly everywhere else in Saranac. In my mother's Santanoni, Ray Brook was spoken of with the same crossed-fingers shudder that children use when they speak of graveyards at Halloween.

Many of the Ray Brook lungers, as they were called, were from the slums of New York City—desperate cases which had become well advanced in crowded conditions where medical attention was not often sought. The doctors whose reputations lent such prestige to the board of trustees at Trudeau did not practice here. The mortality rate of Ray Brook was staggeringly high, perhaps in part because Trudeau, preferring to keep its own slate looking good, shipped its mortally ill patients there. Trudeau maintained that it was not in business to treat terminal cases.

Ray Brook was as completely removed from the village as a leper colony, and its ambulatory patients were forced to find their own amusements on the grounds, with the student nurses or in the nearby speakeasies. Sunday was the big day, when everybody who could get out of bed was allowed to dress and attend church services on the lawn. Never did clergymen speak to such packed audiences—the adage that there are few atheists in foxholes probably applies here—but, more importantly, the men's and women's wards were otherwise well segregated, and the mere idea of dressing up to meet someone of the opposite sex was something to think about all week.

Trudeau Institute, of course, just a stone's throw from Park Avenue, was Valhalla, but you couldn't get in if you were very sick. In the early twenties the famous Institute accepted only the slightest cases because only they were considered worth working on—"after that they were regarded as practically doomed," says an article in its archives. Possibly Trudeau personnel thought of themselves as practicing a kind of triage. In 1926 Trudeau treated 515 patients, of whom 343 were discharged as at least temporarily arrested. If you were accepted at Trudeau, you had real cause for rejoicing. It meant that somebody in the seats of power considered that you had a good chance of pulling through.

In addition, it was a good life, especially considering that it was semi-charitable and the cost (including medical care) neglible, $15 to $24 in the twenties. The patients lived in attractive cottages, most designed by William Scopes, the architect of the Santanoni. From the research conducted in the affiliated Saranac Laboratories issued the best, albeit still meager, information currently available on tuberculosis in the country; and the lab reports on the number of tuberculosis bacilli that could be counted in a sputum sample under a microscope ruled the lives of some of the most envied consumptives in Saranac. A long waiting list of hopefuls was consulted whenever a vacancy occurred.

The fortunate selectees began their stay at the Trudeau Reception and Medical Pavilion, the men on the right and the women the left. Here they awaited results of tests, examination of their chests and X-rays, were assigned a doctor and given a rulebook with a number and a little tin sputum cup to keep by the bed. Through the decades the emphasis changed, but in the twenties the patients spent eight frigid hours out of doors, napped without reading from two to four, returned, if they had exercise permission, to the grounds by 7:30 in the evening and were pulling up the covers by ten. No talk of tuberculosis was allowed in the central dining hall, and visiting between the sexes was limited to an hour and a half in the afternoon, strictly in plain view of everyone on the porch.

Gatherings were occasionally scheduled for the ambulatory—movies, costume balls and skits, most of which revolved around the tyranny of the temperature stick, the timeless elasticity of a cure period and the boredom of so much milk and eggs. Social interchange was built on the base of the things everybody wanted to know about everybody else—how bad is it with you, how long have you been curing and how did you learn you had it? The rest of the time was usually devoted to talking about who had recently "thrown a ruby," the TB slang for a hemorrhage.

All the doctors who followed Trudeau to Saranac took their cures at the Insititute, which alone stamped it as the best care available. While it was cheap, it was not really for the indigent. Titled people sometimes appeared on the rosters, for, like everything else, it was a matter of connections and also of whether or not your condition met the specifications. Acceptance hinged on interesting medical details within certain guidelines.

There were distinguished names in the cottages and also people who, if not for the fact that they were ill, had never had it so good. Like the wartime army, Trudeau living cut across social barriers and made friends of people who would never have met in the worlds from which they came. A high preponderance of medical personnel weighted the patient roster, possibly because the medical profession takes care of its own, but more probably because doctors, nurses and technicians caught the disease often in their line of work.

Trudeau's stringent requirements often separated couples when both members were suffering from the disease. It would accept only those whose condition suited its policy, and the more seriously ill spouses would be left to make other arrangements. The private sanitariums of the village—from the Santanoni and the Altavista to the tiniest hastily swept-out spare room turned into a "cottage san"—catered to those who could not enter Trudeau because either they were too ill or there was no room.

Rich and poor, they kept pouring into the depot down in the village, referred by their home doctors to the famous men, and searching bleakly for a place to stay. Many had no money at all—only a compelling desire to stay in the land of the living. As early as 1907 the doctors gathered together to discuss founding an anti-TB society, one of whose express purposes was to "aid in enforcing sanitary laws, educate people in regard to TB and to spread abroad information that it is futile for a patient to seek any permanent benefits unless he possesses at least $250."

The men of healing had in mind what were locally known as "deadheads," seriously ill patients with no wherewithal whatsoever. In 1927 a man writing to *The Journal of Outdoor Life* complained that, in advance of being weighed, he offered to remove a pocketful of change in the interests of accuracy, but was told to hold on to it, he would need plenty of it in Saranac.

7

The thin, glass-encased column of mercury, which Thomas Mann called the quicksilver cigar, ruled my mother's life as the days blended into each other. Looking at it in the nurse's hand as she shook it down four times a day was like facing an examination for which she could not prepare and which, if she failed, meant corporal punishment. She marveled at the casual way the nurse handled the stick, chatting of trivia, smiling, when its verdict was a matter of living or existing in a vacuum.

She willed her temperature down, forcing herself to relax against the pillow as if not moving would make a difference. She considered sneaking forbidden sips of ice water beforehand, but was afraid to resort to trickery in order to get out of bed. She could think of little else as she waited to hear the next reading, praying for subnormal early-morning temperature so that the inevitable elevation at four would stay below the magic 100 figure. But the infection went on burning in her lung, and her fever chart continued to indicate bed rest.

She did not feel bad. On the contrary, her fever brightened her eyes and quickened her desire for company, for conversation with others besides nurses. She read and reread the letters from her friends at home, bursting with news of parties and small talk calculated to cheer her up but which only succeeded in making her feel left out, buried alive.

The post-hemorrhage lassitude was gone.

Dr. Brown came and went, saying little. She asked to be propped up and wrote a poem or two to her children back in the gray shingle house on Maple Street. Only one letter a day was allowed; the half-finished embroidered guest towels in the basket beside her bed remained forbidden activity— sewing expends nine calories per hour. The days slipped by, her focus on the magic moment in the amorphous future when the thermometer would relax its prohibition and she could join the world.

She came across a poem and kept it to show to the nurse:

> Oh friend; have you not felt the wild desire
> To call your mouth thermometer a liar?

My father came again and again, sitting at the foot of the bed, looking consciously cheerful. He thought she looked better, seemed to have put on weight, but there was something about her that bothered him.

"Do the children miss me?" she wanted to know.

"Bess," he reproved her gently. "Of course."

"But I mean really miss me? Even the baby?"

He nodded.

"Do you think they'll catch it?" she asked, plucking at the blanket. "Or you? You probably ought not to be sitting there. I'm very contagious, you know."

He shook his head and lit a cigarette.

They were bound together by all kinds of strings—a network of love and worry and fear—but they were separate islands. And there were some things about her he did not understand.

"The disease," said Dr. Brown, "is treacherous. The germ slumbers not nor does it sleep."

It sounded Biblical, from some special Bible reserved for consumptives, my mother said, but Dr. Brown only smiled and packed away his stethoscope, saying for the millionth time that she would have to be patient.

The restlessness my mother was displaying was something that Dr. Brown had seen before, again and again and again. Tuberculosis was as double-headed as the jack of spades—on the one hand, it was referred to as the tired disease, and on the other, the fever burning from the lung infection stimulated energy in the frail bodies of the patients which they could ill afford to expend. "Nature has cunningly equipped, for the struggle of life, the little speck of living matter known as the bacillus of TB, which paves the way for its destructive action by stimulating its host to overactivity," wrote Dr. Charles Mayo.

Many consumptives have said that the disease enhanced the colors of life, their perceptions and their personal emotions. Tuberculars often exhibited febrile excitement, a "butterfly within fluttering for release," Elizabeth Barrett Browning called it. The noted writer Katherine Mansfield, identifying the tubercular infection in her doctor, said, "He has the disease himself. I recognize the smile—just the least shade too bright—and his strange joyousness as he came to meet me— the gleam—the faint glitter on the plant that the frost has laid a finger on."

John Keats did his best work while suffering from tuberculosis. Sidney Lanier, the nineteenth-century Southern poet, wrote "Sunrise" when he was near death from the disease. The fever seemed to exist both physically and in the mind. Molière died of consumption almost onstage, driven to the last by the restless urge to continue his work in the teeth of what he must have known was his approaching death.

The doctors recognized this characteristic of TB even while they imperfectly understood the disease. Some said it was the outgrowth of increased mental activity stimulated by constant rest and the fear of death. Others said it was due to actual toxic agents manufactured by the TB bacilli and spilled into the nervous system. Twenty years after the onset of my mother's illness they were still wrestling with this problem, studying the nervous irritability and enormous drive which could be medically documented in patients and which many compared to working under the influence of alcohol or narcotics.

John Addington Symonds said that tuberculosis gave him a wonderful "Indian summer of experience." Ralph Waldo Emerson, who also had it, put it differently. "A mouse," he said, "is gnawing at my chest."

Dr. Maurice Fishberg was quoted as late as 1940 as saying that "many tubercular patients show a remarkable change in their mental traits and characteristics, a disturbance in the emotional life and a striking divergence from their previous habits, affections and tastes."

The patient, says Dr. G. M. Munro in his book on the

psychopathology of tuberculosis, has an insatiable craving for life.

The light burned too brightly, and the tuberculars reacted in various ways.

In many, the false energy, coupled with the eagerness to seize the fleeting moments in the teeth of possible death, found its outlet in the sexual stimulation which tubercular patients widely experienced. Oblique references to this phenomenon can be found in textbooks of the period, usually explained as the outgrowth of the damaging of the nervous system by germs and the close proximity of people with like problems and nothing to do but lie in bed. Whatever is was, it was a fact of life. "You're not married after you leave Utica," was the adage of the twenties in Saranac Lake, and there were plenty of data to back it up.

What did my mother feel, lying there in the first months of her stay in Saranac? Whatever she did feel was filtered out of her letters home and, for all I know, from what she said to my father. Did she worry that her marriage would founder, as so many did under months, years of separation? Did she worry that my father would find it too easy to become the perennial extra man while she lay day after day in her bed? Barely thirty, not sure that she would live to know whatever there was left to discover in the world, did she have to push down the fear that her sexual life was over?

I don't know. My parents were private people. Even years later they would not have thought of mentioning such a thing, nor would their friends after they were both dead. Even now I feel uneasy considering it. I never saw my father so much as kiss my mother or heard him call her by an endearment, though he loved her dearly.

My father told me much, much later that hostesses called

him constantly, and he must have gone, for I do not think he was a man who cared to be lonely and I remember him only occasionally eating with us children. He was married, but he was not married. It must have been a difficult time, but he never spoke of it.

Elsewhere in Saranac Lake things were different.

"You were building up your health and you were just lying there," says a man who took the cure a bit later. "And some of the women patients were available—it was a game. And the student nurses were drawn to the patients and the drama of it all. There was regular traffic after lights out up the hill to the nurses' dorm and elsewhere in the dark."

"Cousining" was the word they used. No matter how married you were, it was different in Saranac. There might not be a tomorrow—everybody in the line of beds knew that—and your former life was as remote as if it had taken place in China. Right beside you were people who understood this and had exactly the same problems. Everybody had a cousin.

At Trudeau the little rustic gazebos were favorite rendezvous spots for the ambulatory, and the village still refers to them as cousinolas. They were not very private—a roof and a railing—but they were better than a sleeping porch.

"Of course you thought quite a while before you gave a girl with tuberculosis a good kiss on the mouth," says the same man.

But they did. It was all part of the pattern of the disease, the bed rest, the close proximity, the desire, the need for love and reassurance that you were not, after all, damaged goods. The need for human warmth when you didn't know if you would ever re-enter the world.

It took hold of people who would not otherwise have considered having an affair, people whose religion, background and heritage normally would have forbidden such behavior.

One man recounts that he fell into a liaison with a pretty Italian girl curing at Ray Brook whose husband ran a movie theater in Brooklyn. She had never undressed before her husband, nor would he have considered such a thing. But in her new affair she was absolutely uninhibited. With death looking over her shoulder, she threw away the rulebook, forgot the reserve that had held her back all her life, gave herself up in abandon. For months they carried on a tender and deeply passionate sexual relationship.

She was one of the lucky ones who recovered and went back home. The man with whom she was involved never heard from her again—with the exception of a single phone call. Over the wires from Brooklyn she whispered that she had reverted to her old reserve, that sex was no longer a sinless joy. The fever was over. It was like a page turned forever.

This was, apparently, far from rare. Ray Brook rules were extremely strict, but there was no way to check on everybody. Every night they stole out in the dead of the night, met a taxi parked on the side road which would carry them to a tryst. Tomorrow it might be too late, and, while they could, they would not hold back.

It was not usually indiscriminate. Your cousin was your steady. They were intense, burning love affairs, not always consummated, partly because of lack of opportunity and partly because of the ever-present worry that exertion would overtax the healing. But always it was a relationship you could lean on so that what happened back home would be bearable if it turned out, as it often did, badly. One of the most common sights in Saranac was the weekend visit of a spouse while the cousin sat glowering in the background, without the right to speak.

Many, of course, never came to visit their sick spouses, but after having delivered them to the sanitarium, drove away figuratively dusting their hands. Loose ties, financial strain—many marriages could not sustain such separations and such deprivations as the long cures demanded. Cousining was the most natural thing in the world, and it made the whole thing more bearable.

Disrupted marriages were common even if the sick partner got well. Taking the cure put a lifelong stamp on you. The pace became ingrained, the push of life elsewhere looked frighteningly brisk from Saranac, many of the old jobs were too demanding and suggested too many possibilities of relapse, the old fear of cured tuberculars. With their old life in shambles, many recovered patients stayed on, having nothing to go back to or preferring what they had. Tuberculosis was a great common denominator, and Saranac today is full of people who came from Brooklyn, Hartford, Montreal, Boston, Glens Falls and elsewhere and remained to make a life where they were understood.

"Were you sick?" they ask each other on the streets.

"Of course. Who wasn't?"

The nurses felt the tide of desperate lovemaking more than any others. They were inevitably drawn to their patients, in spite of, or maybe because of, the danger. Many were men of education and position who had gained assurance from their success, and the nurses were in daily contact with them. Some of the nurses got so thoroughly involved that they tried to commit suicide.

The nurses who had had affairs with patients were the

ones the Saranac Lotharios were especially cautious about kissing.

The town's hot spots were full of cousining couples: Downing and Carie, a bar and restaurant whose prices were possible for financially embarrassed patients; Hennesey's bar; the Barn in Lake Placid, where the more affluent took their cousins to hold hands and whisper over the meal.

The nineteenth century saw consumptives as romantic, wan and wasting, marked for an early grave, but interesting as they feverishly burned themselves out writing novels and poetry. But the early part of the twentieth century understood consumption to be dangerously contagious and its cure only a possibility. Thus, its victims fell from their romanticized pedestal to a position not unlike that of the leper. Under the circumstances, its victims did what they could with the life their ostracization left them.

8

By Christmas my mother was improving. The little radio by her bed, which up to now had been silent, rattled on hour after hour, and Dr. Brown had lifted the restrictions on her reading. The guest towels had finally come out of their basket, though it was hard for her to see to work on them in a semi-recumbent position. Most exciting of all, more earth-shaking than a revolution in China, was the new permission to take the few steps to the bathroom every other day.

It was the tiniest of liberties, but it represented giant progress. To feel the carpet once more beneath her feet, to view the world from a vertical position, however transitorily, was heady. Her spirits improved as if she had been let out of jail. Once more she was looking outward to the world beyond her suite, asking my father if the nurse was pretty, if he had many invitations to dinner. When he recounted how, at the last party, the host had run out of gin and disappeared upstairs to concoct more, she laughed.

It had been a long time since she had laughed.

Christmas Day she sat for the first time in her reclining chair for an hour, her lap full of presents and her eyes full of tears. There would be no presents from her under the tree at home for us children, and she would not be there to see our faces as we watched the real little candles on every branch lit. My brother, who was already seven, would not understand her absence. Her red velvet dress would stay in the closet. In the prettily wrapped packages on her lap were bed jackets and soft woolly throws for her cure chair and bed.

Every day they rolled her out onto her sleeping porch, where she could watch the snow coming down so thickly it was like one of the paperweights the children upended to make a Christmas scene out of the little figures in the glass dome. She lay, hot-water bottle at her feet, wrapped in a horse blanket which they had put on the mattress and pulled back over her regular bedclothing to enclose her like the contents of an envelope. Even with the hot-water bottle, her feet grew cold, and my father brought a pair of bed socks, full of mistakes, which her closest friend had knitted. She wore deerskin gloves lined in fur which made it difficult to turn the pages of her book.

The long hours oozed into each other, each like the one before, as she lay watching the snow drift on the mountains and trying not to cough. They were stern about coughing.

"You don't scratch every itch," the nurses said, smiling to show they weren't really cross. But all around her she could hear the others coughing on their porches—deep, loose coughs with a frightening rattle in them. It takes energy to cough, they told her, energy you need to get well. They told her about the patient who had suggested that the cough power of the million-plus tuberculars in the country might be harnessed to produce something useful like the building of the Panama Canal.

She did not smile. The snow continued, and when at last it stopped, the cold intensified so that the very air seemed to crackle. Frost glittered on the tops of the cars in the street below, and the people, picking their way slowly and carefully through the shoveled-out streets, looked like bundled-up bears. When the sun shone, the glare was blinding. A million diamonds reflected off the scene below her porch and, when she shut her eyes, danced inside her lids. She worked her way for the second time through *Nicholas Nickleby* and *Our Mutual Friend,* and the days dragged on.

And then one day Dr. Brown said she could get dressed. Get dressed and go down to dinner.

It was the one thing that she had longed for, counted the hours till, and when it came she was afraid. It was like a commuted life sentence, but it was also like a dangerous expedition alone through the wilderness. She had lain in the bed too long. Now that she could leave it for a few hours, bed seemed a small, safe kingdom. Outside there would be new people, strangers. She was at once drunk with happiness and as timid as she had ever been in her life.

Watching her face, Dr. Brown's own grew grave.

"You must not overdo," he warned. "It's so easy at this stage. If you feel the least tired, stop. If your temperature goes back up over ninety-nine point five, it's back into the cure chair and bed all day."

The threat of recall banished the timidity. When the nurses

came, she told them the news. It was like coming home from school with a good report, and they patted her shoulder and twittered about her like birds. They had told her all along, had they not, that this day would come?

But of course she must be careful. Dressing is exercise, they said sternly. It must be taken in easy stages. And if she was to go down to dinner that very day, now she must rest. Just see, they said, pointing to the empty streets outside the window without so much as a small boy on a sled: the whole of Saranac was resting, and so must she.

She scarcely heard what they were saying. She was trying to decide what to wear.

When the lights of the village were just beginning to come on, they chose the black chiffon with the handkerchief hemline which had been hanging unused in the back of the closet. They knelt to find the little black silk shoes with the pointed toes and the rhinestone buckles. They eased the dress over her head as carefully as if they were dressing a doll. It was dangerous to raise the arms: the cavity must not be disturbed.

She had gained weight, and the dress was tight. It pulled over the hips, and she frowned in front of the long glass, but emancipation outweighed what she saw in her reflection. They helped her dress her hair, poufed the pompadour with the little rat of combings kept in the silver box on the bureau. She took her little bag with her handkerchief and her cigarette holder and she was ready to step into the elevator which had delivered her to her room so many weeks ago.

It descended slowly, opening its doors at length into a pleasant lobby which she had scarcely noticed when she arrived. A turn to the left and she was in the dining room, a handsome paneled room with a big bay window overlooking the village and the long drive up from Church Street.

A new ambulatory patient made heads turn all over the

room. Smart-looking women in evening gowns—to dress at all was so exciting that only the very best would do—men in dinner jackets. They absorbed her at once in the friendliest possible way, offering her a seat, inquiring which was her doctor and how long she had been on bed rest. To be in this dining room was to be friends with them at once. She felt at last part of it all, escaped from her solitary cocoon.

Lovely food, but she could not eat a bite. It was all too exciting, and the courses arrived and were removed while she compared notes with the woman on her right and the distinguished-looking gentleman across.

"But you must eat," they admonished her, and she nodded and picked at the chocolate éclair. They invited her to join them at the bridge table, but she was suddenly as tired as she had ever been in all her life. Her legs felt like jelly, and when the elevator opened its door to her once again, she stepped thankfully in, promising to meet them all again tomorrow.

Like sisters after a party, the nurses helped her undress, and she fell into bed and slept as she had not slept for months.

It is not so long ago, but how archaic it sounds: the long weeks in bed and then the slow, careful, step-at-a-time journey back into the normal world. Wonder drugs have accustomed us to miracles; the twenties had none. To overdo was to begin the whole process all over again, and the prohibitions were removed so gradually it sometimes took years. Some made the gradual, careful climb back to normalcy, treading carefully lest they awaken the sleeping germs, and some repeatedly returned to their bed with fever. There was no magic pill, no healing panacea. The doctors could see Koch's red-stained bacillus in the microscopic slides, but they had no real weapons to deal with it.

For centuries the disease had puzzled the physicians. Tuberculosis may well have been the first of the pestilences, for exhumed skeletons from prehistoric periods bear its marks. Treatment from the very beginning was hit-or-miss. In the court of Louis XIV, quinine and tar water were a favorite remedy. Others administered milk from an ass which had received forty inunctions of mercury. Or the bark of Peru, or digitalis, or bouillon made from the lungs of a viper or a calf.

In the twenties the doctors were still interested in the lungs of a calf, but for somewhat more enlightened reasons. They were always searching for the one treatment which could change the course of history, heal lungs which were riddled with cavities, pocked with abcesses. Morris Dworski, later director of the chemical lab at the Will Rogers Sanitarium in Saranac, where the entertainment world cured, remembers Dr. Kinghorn calling him on the telephone and announcing excitedly: "Morris, I have a cow's lung in the bathtub. You'd better come right over."

What they did with it is not recorded. But other attempts to short-circuit the long weeks in bed failed miserably. At one time the doctors attempted to plug the yawning cavities clearly visible in the X-rays of consumptive lungs with wax. But the wax melted, and the idea was abandoned in favor of filling the chest surgically with Ping-Pong balls, which would squeeze the lung into submissive rest. They still speak in awe in the streets of Saranac Lake of the man who had 112 Ping-Pong balls in his chest. He survived the operation for three years and became a familiar figure in Saranac, walking as if his chest were full of lead instead of plastic. It was not much of a life.

Inevitably the doctors also tried the chemical route. The

Addiline Medical Company of Columbus, Ohio, manufactured a germicide which it claimed killed germ growth in the tubercular lung. The Saranac laboratories analyzed it and found that the medicine consisted largely of oils, petroleum and pine, and such aromatic herbs as thyme.

Said Dr. Edward R. Baldwin, director, who spoke with all the majesty of Trudeau Institute behind him: "The effect of these oils on tuberculosis would of course be fatal and the cleverness of the originator is shown in this way . . . if you can catch a flea and put powder on him, you can certainly commit homicide! The same thing might happen to the tuberculosis bacillus if he should happen to fall into this Addiline oil."

The pungent liquid was apt to cause belching, and the Addiline company handily made an asset out of this by claiming that this was even better because one then breathed the fumes a second time.

Down through the ages the medical men had searched for a cure and failed. Cod-liver oil was once the standard remedy, and as late as the fifties it was still given as a vitamin supplement to bolster the body in its difficult struggle with the germs. But most of the remedies were aimed at alleviating the symptoms of the disease, much as aspirin and liquids such as fruit juices or tea give symptomatic relief for a cold. It made the patients feel better to sniff herbs; sucking ice sometimes kept them from coughing blood; and opium, first tested in the Hôpital de la Charité in Paris, made them believe for a short happy period that they were better.

During the early nineteenth century European and English physicians observed that citizens of warm climates often got tuberculosis when they migrated to colder regions, so it was deduced that the most salubrious climate for tuberculosis was a mild one. Monkeys were especially prone to develop tuberculosis in the cold, damp climate of England after living most of their lives in the branches of a tropical banyan tree. The medical men reasoned that cold climates meant more risk of consumption, which was both true and erroneous. The truth was that, whether monkeys or men, those who came or were brought to cold climates encountered for the first time the consumption germs to which the natives had developed some immunity and were more likely to fall victim because they had not previously been exposed.

The idea that a mild climate was important treatment for weak lungs persisted far into the nineteenth century. Sir James Clare, physician to Keats in Rome and later to Queen Victoria, recommended the climate of Rome and the Riviera. For those who found it hard to come by the necessary money to get to those cities, he suggested purchasing a special stove and keeping the windows closed except for a few minutes each day.

Bed rest for consumptives in the twenties probably had its beginning in the early vogue for sea voyages for those in delicate health. The idea of lying about languidly in a deck chair was first cousin to the enforced bed rest my mother and her contemporaries had to endure. On the other hand, in the seventeenth century long horseback rides were suggested for sufferers from lung complaints. A leisurely foray in the saddle was considered at that time to be as good as lounging in your favorite chair and had the advantage of keeping one in the open air. Many European doctors of the period suggested that their tubercular patients secure jobs as coachmen.

Tuberculosis was, for some time, without doubt the greatest killer in the Western world, and many died from it whose deaths appeared on medical records attributed to bronchitis, gastric fever, scrofula or asthenia. Sometimes the illness was merely referred to as "going into a decline," a phrase implying all the preordination of the stars. Some who had it concealed it rather than submit to the inevitable incarceration in a sanitarium, and often the lucky ones who recovered and made their way back into the normal world never spoke of it again. It was a disease whose name, with its implication of death, was whispered behind doors, and it is not really surprising that the cure was long in coming.

Even if the specialists had had any real weapons against TB, the death rate would still have been considerable because the disease, as in my mother's case, was often misdiagnosed. Most frequently it was mistaken for a bad cold that hung on, but many who simply complained of being tired were treated with tonics and various nostrums guaranteed to give them more energy until a pulmonary hemorrhage unmasked the real culprit. Even then, in the early years of this century, the medical men sometimes missed the cue.

John Lathrop, writing in *Collier's Weekly* in 1913 about his own experiences, tells a story which was probably repeated often about the country. He, like so many before and after him, complained to his doctor of fatigue. Though tuberculosis was then the leading cause of death, his doctor, a personal friend, examined him and recommended that he cease worrying about his work and go out and physically tire himself. In view of the prevailing idea of the time that complete rest was almost the only answer to consumption, it makes one shudder to hear how he followed his friend's orders.

"Walk from five to twenty miles a day, or climb a mountain every day or do at least half a man's work on a farm," advised his doctor friend. "Get tired. Get so tired that you drop asleep every night the moment you hit the pillow."

Lathrop did as he was told, but, not surprisingly, did not improve.

"Then one night," says Lathrop, ". . . I awoke at about eleven o'clock at night, terrified with a sensation I had never experienced before. The inclination to cough was strong, [yet] instinct commanded me not to yield if it lay within my human power to resist successfully. As the moments passed and I fought that terrible fight, it came over me, swiftly, yet surely, that I was threatened with a pulmonary hemorrhage. Ignorant as I was, I nevertheless reasoned that if possible I should prevent that cough from agitating my frame. So I summoned every whit of will power, held myself rigid, controlled my throat muscles, breathed with enough inspiration to bring just a trifle of air into my lungs and fought, fought, fought as the precious moments fled.

". . . against my most extreme resistance a slight cough shook me and a . . . hemorrhage followed."

At last suspecting tuberculosis, Lathrop and his wife summoned a new doctor to examine him. The second medical man pronounced the blood of no consequence, a nasal phenomenon, and told him he was quite fit to go on a business trip he was planning the following morning. Something told the poor man that he was not, and he remained at home, where he suffered a second hemorrhage. Then, and only then, was tuberculosis diagnosed.

The disease seems to have been astonishingly difficult for the doctors of the period to diagnose, and at least as difficult, except in light cases, to cure. This being the case, the doctors offered palliatives, high on the list of which was thinking cheerful thoughts. Possibly the patients with the best chance of recovery were quite naturally more cheerful than others, and so the doctors, mistaking cause and effect, began to regard optimism as a requisite of getting well. They also believed that despair used up more ergs than a positive attitude, and lacking better weapons, they pushed good cheer.

Straight into the twenties the medical men clung to this belief in the power of optimism. Thus, the doctors nodded in approval when a group of Jewish patients in Trudeau obediently formed a Good Cheer Club. *The Journal Of Outdoor Life* during the twenties is larded with inspirational quotes lifted from the writings of famous men and from the pens of patients having nothing much better to do. In the face of the startling mortality figures of the day—121,500 died from tuberculosis in the United States in 1920 alone—the consumptives had precious little to hold on to except their will to live. Lacking any alternative, they adjured each other to "Buck up and cheer up," a motto selected by the consumptives' official magazine.

"Doctors," says a letter to the *Saranac Lake News* in the twenties, "we're all chipped and broken pottery here, but we rattle around and make a cheerful noise."

In the annals of Trudeau it is nevertheless recorded that a nurse was let go from the staff because too many complained about her excessive cheerfulness.

With what tools they had, the physicians of the twenties worked diligently to help the consumptives, but were only too aware that they would not always be successful.

The inscription on Dr. Edward Trudeau's statue has an oddly hedging ring:

> To cure sometimes
> To relieve often
> To comfort always.

9

If the town outside my mother's windows at the Santanoni
was as hectic as a frontier town, the pace inside was deliberately slowed to the kind of progress one makes when attempting to walk underwater. Time was stretched and elongated
until it was as meaningless as it seems after an anesthetic. It
existed on several levels, in different layers for different
patients, but for none did it have any definite outline. The
present was a holding operation for the future, when all the
good things of life would happen. In the meantime, one could
think about it, plan, make arrangements. Even these were
done in slow motion—next week was precipitously near to
plan for; two or three weeks gave one time to think and for

details to fall into place. Meanwhile, there was much to be discussed.

My mother's isolation was over. Like soldiers in the army, all patients were friends. There was none of the preliminary feeling out, that cautious sounding which precedes friendship in ordinary life. They had the same problems and the same doctors, and they accepted each other instantly. It was as if they had always known each other.

Of course the Santanoni patients were in various stages of cure, and my mother met only those allowed to come down for meals. Many of these were on exercise and would come by to chat of a morning, bringing her treasures from the village— the latest best-seller, a tin of butterscotch, some pears from Charlie Green's fruit store. They assured her that they had once been confined as she was now, and only see how they had improved and were allowed out. It cheered her vastly, and she liked them all.

Then there was the day that Adrian and Henry, friends from Rome, came rolling up the long drive to visit. Adrian sat ramrod straight in the easy chair, reporting everything that had happened in the time since she had been gone, and Henry said she looked far healthier than anyone at home. She introduced them to her new friend Mrs. Diat, who was doing so well she was already on exercise. They had brought a thermos of Manhattan cocktails because Henry had a very trusty bootlegger, and my father said this came under the heading of coals to Newcastle. It was like old times, with everyone laughing and talking at the same time.

Of course it tired her. They were the first official visitors, and she lay all day in the cure chair the next day, feeling as if she had climbed Mount McKenzie, at which she was getting very tired of looking. But her fever stayed low, and a few weeks later Dr. Brown allowed her to go down to both lunch and dinner and then to breakfast. To say goodbye to the tray after so many interminable months was heady, but they warned her to move slowly, to walk as she had seen the others walking, using what they called the TB tread, which reminded her of an old movie slowed down for a moment to savor a scene that is especially delightful.

For my mother, a woman who up to now had hurried through life, it was alien, and she felt like a colt being broken to bridle. But she did what they said because she was afraid not to. And, anyway, everybody else walked the same way.

She was invited to play bridge in the morning and also after the sacrosanct nap, when no deliveries were accepted and small boys were forbidden their bicycles. She was asked for more bridge after dinner, and as she gradually improved, she accepted. They were very good players and knew all the latest rules, so she boned up in her room so that she shouldn't disgrace herself.

She was not yet on exercise, but, listening to the chatter, she knew it would not now be long. She was following the prescribed pattern, step by step; they had all been there before her. And it would be so gay. They were always driving off somewhere in a group—she felt quite left out—in a taxi to the Pontiac to see the latest film, over to Placid to see the skaters, to Lower Saranac Lake to have a picnic at a camp they'd rented.

There were others who were not even allowed out of their beds after months, but she did not know them, though her new friends shook their heads sadly when they spoke of them. But then they would cheer up and plan another sleigh ride or expedition to watch the curling. It was all approved by the doctors, including Dr. Brown.

"The current popular belief in Saranac Lake," he said, "is that one hour of driving is worth two of sitting on the porch."

Any time they weren't actually doing these things, they were planning them. Would So-and-so, who had recently had a setback and higher fever, be well enough to go? Should they engage a guide to build a fire and fry some of the lake fish which he would provide, or should they be content to take chicken sandwiches and hot soup, with perhaps some fruit and pastries they would tease from the chef? Each detail must be considered, and the pros and cons took up hours of their time.

She longed to go with them, to sit beside Mrs. Diat in the big sleigh they were planning to engage for a night ride to Placid, to sing all the way with them, though she could not carry a tune—in the frigid, brittle, crystal cold under the stars as the horses' hooves clip-clopped along the road in the shadow of the mountains. But Dr. Brown was not to be hurried. It was too soon, he said, and in the meantime she was never to stand when she could sit, never to sit when she could lie.

She felt like a piece of fragile china. She pouted, but it was fun just to listen to them. Long before she set foot on Main Street or Broadway, she knew everything about the village.

They gossiped over the cards. They knew just who was having an affair with whom and what movie about the Canadian Mounties was being made up at Moody's Pond at Caribou Bill's movie camp. They knew who had coughed sputum flecked with blood, and when Irvin S. Cobb was visiting Carl Palmer up at 135 Park. One of them was sure to have spotted Paul Whiteman's Cunningham parked down on Broadway, and somebody always had a story to tell about Gonzales Cottage, where the Spanish patients mostly cured.

They knew when Mme. Schumann-Heink was scheduled to sing under the auspices of the Tuberculosis Society and what kind of fish they were having for dinner.

For they lived, all of them, in a never-never land, a between-and-betwixt place where few were mortally ill but no one at all was well. And everyone had plenty of everything except health, and what they most especially had was time. And since not one of them could plan his life, which was dependent on the doctors' verdict, they had to be content with thinking about next month.

They drank cocktails, murmuring that alcohol stimulated the appetite and they were only attempting to please Dr. Trembley or Dr. Mayer or Dr. Welles. Someone was always asking two or three in for sherry in his living room before dinner, and that was a party too. Everyone looked well dressed and ready to be amused; some of the women even smoked, holding their long cigarette holders casually and dribbling ashes as they recounted their temperature charts. They tried not to talk about their disease, but somehow it always came around to that. It knit them together, as expatriates are knit together when they meet in foreign countries.

They looked well, most of them, though some were still trying to cover too prominent hipbones and sunken chests with fat. My mother's own face had filled out, and everyone complimented her on her looks. They thought she must be doing well, pausing gracefully to hear what Dr. Brown had said, because several also had Dr. Brown and wanted to compare notes.

But the evenings were early, and then there was too much time to think about the future and the meaning of life. Tuberculosis is an introspective disease, and time abounded. In spite of herself, my mother would let the book fall into her lap as she lay in bed, losing the thread of the narrative at the thought of the months slipping by, months which made huge differences in young children and in her own youth. And then she would get the feeling that the whole world was rushing on and that she was in a backwater from which she could not escape, and she would fall into a black mood. And before it was time to turn out the light, she would write yet another letter to my father reminding him to see that my brother got a haircut and to tell Kathleen that she must iron my dresses with the smocking with a cool iron from the wrong side.

And in spite of the progress that Dr. Brown said he thought she was making, and the new friends and the sleigh rides to come, she still felt like an exile.

"You must bring the children to see me soon," she wrote firmly at the bottom of the letter. "We will be careful."

The sense of isolation which my mother felt must have been multiplied a hundredfold for many of the patients in the nearby sanitariums, including the "up cottages," where the patients were ambulatory. It made an expedition into town seem as important and exciting as a safari to Africa. Many had not heard from their families in months, had left large cities where they had respected niches, busy lives, and family ties, and often where the outdoors was something they looked at through a window. Now their base was a bed on a sleeping porch and their future questionable at best. It is remarkable that so many bore with good grace the long weeks in bed, the strict prohibitions, the lack of definite prognosis and the ostracism from normal life.

The periodicals of the time were full of the bad poetry and peptalk for consumptives written by other consumptives. For example:

Another year! My, how you fret!
Your lungs are far from perfect yet.
You're certain as you dry your tears
The Doc said months, he sure meant years.

In 1930 a woman patient, despairing of the consumptive life, lay down on the railroad track near the bridge at Moody's Pond and let the train from Lake Placid run over her; lying on the track, she had waited while the train whistled a last-ditch warning from a mile away. The furor the incident caused makes it clear that few took this route, and it would be difficult to establish that the suicide rate for tuberculosis was anything to remark on.

Yet the boredom warred strangely with the fear of death, the shadow of which lurked in the future of every consumptive. The mortality rate of tuberculosis at the time might be compared to the death rate for cancer patients today, but the psyche of the victims was different. There was no pain, and the very treatment of the disease itself did not encourage dramatic decisions. Leafing through the logbooks of the Fortune and Keough funeral homes for the period, one can see how many died every day. Yet they seemed to wait it out with a soldier's fatalism laced with a dash of Foreign Legion desperate bravado. The total despair of a patient informed he has cancer would have been alien to Saranac Lake.

For these patients were trying to get well. It was a competitive game, and, wherever they came from, Saranac became the center of their universe. An Adirondack village two minutes from the wilderness, it rearranged itself around their needs, catered to them, waited on them, took care of them, sometimes bilked them.

It takes no imagination to see Saranac Lake as it was in the twenties, when tuberculosis was the country's most feared disease and tuberculars filled the narrow streets, taking their exercise allotment attired in wool underwear (very scratchy), wool ski pants and raccoon and opossum coats. It all is still there, like Pompeii preserved in ash, for after the miracle drugs were discovered, the health seekers departed leaving everything just as it was. Everything that hasn't burned down remains—the old hotels, the railroad station, the lavish brown-shingled private residences, creosoted to stand the winters, the little houses with stuck-on sleeping porches, the Pontiac Theatre with its garish green-and-silver front and the hole in the sidewalk where a chain once held back the crowds eager for entertainment. Dr. Trudeau's neat red home is just as he left it at the corner of Church and Main—his grandson practices general medicine in his office—and the Hotel Saranac still takes in paying guests.

Everything is as if they had only gone yesterday, taking the last train from the lovely old station with its domed cupola and peaked roof—or driving off in their old high Packards, finally given permission to leave their beds. It is like a battlefield after the armistice, the contestants gone and the site unchanged and abandoned.

But of course they didn't all go. Many of them are still there; in the outer office of the *Adirondack Enterprise,* which they used to call the "Empty Prize," living in dark apartments over the Pontiac Theatre on Broadway, or down Main Street in the shadow of the Hotel Saranac.

And in St. Bernard's cemetery, section D, where they put the bodies of so many who lost the fight.

Or in Pine Ridge cemetery, where more than forty Ray Brook patients sleep forever, buried by the state of New York because their relatives never appeared to claim their bodies.

❧ 10

I think it was close to a year before my father brought us children to see my mother in her apartment at the Santanoni. I have no memory of that first visit, and my brother falls silent when I ask about it. He was going on eight at the time, a solemn little dark-haired boy in a sailor suit. I have seen the pictures of us at this age, me sitting on the step beside him, gazing up at him adoringly from under a big, frilly hat.

I have no memory of the visit, but I know, for I remember later trips, that we stayed well on our side of the room and that I felt on display and shy. The lady lying in the cure chair smiling at me was called Mother. Everyone had made that clear. But I did not know her.

It was not that she hadn't written me carloads of letters which my nurse had read to me, chatty little letters signed with X marks for kisses at the bottom. I knew her as the author of these letters and as a voice on the telephone to which I could not respond, being struck dumb by the enormity of the moment. She was my mother, I knew it, but it was only with Anna, my snowy-haired, pink-cheeked nurse with the generous waistline and prim ways, that I felt comfortable.

There is no way I can tell what we said to each other, we virtual strangers across that small apartment living room, my hand clutched firmly in my father's. There is no way of knowing. I can only put myself, years later, in her place and imagine with what pain she must have viewed someone else bringing up her children. "The baby speaks," she said once later in my hearing to my father, "exactly like Nettie." Nettie was the second maid and a special favorite of mine.

She must have felt cheated, looking at us across the room, but I cannot say for sure, for in those days and in my parents' circle such things were never said aloud, particularly before the children. Whatever disaster befell, a united front of business as usual was always preserved for the children's sake, a studied conspiracy to protect our childhood and keep us from worrying. As a result, in private I worried constantly.

Only here and there did the doors to what they were really thinking swing open briefly for a peep—when they forgot we were there, forgot to smooth things out, to wrap what they felt in proper, ordinary-sounding words.

They were talking of heaven.

This in itself was enough to make me look up from dressing my doll. It was not their kind of conversation. Heaven was mentioned only in prayers. They were considering what heaven might be like, and my mother was asking my father if he thought it was possible to get a clear view over the edge of the clouds to what was going on in the world one had left behind. She was asking if he thought one could develop a viewpoint detached enough to make such an omnipotent knowledge a boon and not a burden.

They tossed the idea about for some time, half laughing, half serious, while I, unnoticed, hung on their words.

My mother finally shook her head.

"No," she said to my father, "it just couldn't be. Because if I die, you will marry again and your new wife might be mean to Betty and I could see it and feel bad. What kind of a heaven would that be?"

It had never occurred to me that she might die, might cease to be my mother, but now, looking at her over my doll's head, I considered the possibility. She was laughing again, but I knew what lay ahead. I could see her lying white and cold in the bed while my brother and I gathered near, weeping.

It was years before I fully understood how intimately a consumptive in the twenties lived with the idea of death and the possibility of contributing to the alarming statistics.

As I look back now across the decades to that first visit to the Santanoni, it is not hard to imagine what she must have thought, seeing her family lined up against the wall. We were her children and she scarcely knew us. And though the fever charts were down, it was common knowledge that they often went up again.

She must have been aware that it was possible she would never be able to put her arms around us again lest she jeopardize our future. It was well documented that children were far more susceptible to TB than adults. The best thing she could do for us was to stay safely across the room. I imagine she smiled at us and inquired after Anna.

We did not come again, I think, for several months.

My mother's problem was shared by many all over the Switzerland of America. Tuberculosis was far more likely to strike the young with families than any other group, and the attendant difficulties were varying. Many of the rich who were not too desperately ill took houses for the duration of their cure, sending their children to the private Baldwin School in the village. Here they mingled with the children of the affluent natives and became their friends, attended their birthday parties, visited them after school. But when it was their turn, it was understood that their homes on Park Avenue were out of bounds. Instead, they entertained their schoolmates at the Pines Club, the private club to which the doctors and the wealthiest patients belonged, or rented a camp on Lower Saranac where the party could be held without fear of contagion.

Saranac was well aware of the special danger to children. Every child in the public schools of the village was, as a matter of course, X-rayed yearly. A $50 fine was imposed and strictly enforced on anyone careless enough to spit in the public streets—and $50 was money then. Saranac knew all too well how easy it was to catch tuberculosis.

For families of patients who could afford to replace absent parents with nurses, tuberculosis was bad enough, but hundreds of others with tiny children had no place to leave them and no money to hire help, and were forced to bring them to Saranac. Marshall McClintock, who wrote a book about his cure in Saranac in the twenties, says that both he and his wife were consumptive and had no choice but to bring their son of toddling age with them. They found successive women willing to care for him for small sums, but most turned out to be either careless or uncaring. At one time they even took an apartment, hoping to keep him with them, though they had to abandon the idea because the care was far too much for their strength. At one time they retrieved the child from a woman who had allowed him to become black with his own excrement, covered with sores, thin and miserable. One of the most touching parts of McClintock's account is the pride with which both he and his wife realized that, in such an uncertain existence, the baby continued to recognize them.

The separations and the expenses are dreadful to contemplate from our world safely hedged about with miracle drugs and insurance policies, but they pale beside the constant presence of fear which was a daily fact of life. The fear came in assorted shapes and colors—fear for one's own life, fear for the children and worry over the friends worse off than oneself. It was all neatly packaged in a frightening cloak of half-knowledge, for as the doctors did not really have many weapons for the cure, neither were they quite sure exactly how the disease was transmitted.

Everyone, of course, understood that coughing spread the germs, which lingered in the room for three hours and projected three feet from the cougher's mouth. But the germs were also transmitted from spit in the streets, brought indoors on shoes or long skirts, where they set up housekeeping and, according to Dr. Brown's handbook, were redistributed when the maid swept. As early as 1920 the doctors had figured out that if you lay on a couch which a tubercular had just vacated, you ran a risk of infection. But no one really knew why some resisted the obviously frequent exposure and remained healthy, and others, living under sanitary and affluent conditions, succumbed. There are some who say now that the peak of mortality for tuberculosis in the twenties was simply a world epidemic abetted by World War I, but there is no real way of knowing now, as there was not then. And so the fear grew.

Dr. Francis Trudeau, grandson of the founder of Trudeau, in his doctoral thesis for Yale on Saranac says that in 1926 there were two beds in every room in the cottage sanitariums. By 1930 this was not allowed, for some patients were far worse off than others. The *How to Get Well Book,* written by a former patient in Trudeau in 1906, warns the reader not to get too involved with fellow patients confined to their rooms and, when moving into a sanitarium, to see that the room is fumigated and scrubbed with disinfectant. If the patients themselves were warned to beware of each other, it is not surprising that the outside world preferred to stay as far away from virulent cases as possible.

Nobody wanted any contact with tuberculosis which could possibly be avoided. In 1920, in a leaflet describing the disease, the New York State Department of Health in Albany took congnizance of this and lamented.

"Considering the natural and acquired resistance to infection which is unquestionably preserved by adults," says the booklet, *What You Should Know About Tuberculosis,* "much unreasonable fear of the disease or phthisiophobia has prevailed in late years. The results of this have sometimes been a deplorable neglect or persecution of tuberculosis patients. Because there is no precaution too great for the protection of the young and delicate, this does not justify healthy adults in exaggerated fears for their own safety."

The fear was especially strong in the people who knew the most about the disease and had seen its effects.

Bill McLaughlin, who used to work for the *Adirondack Enterprise* and later switched to the *Lake Placid News,* says as a boy he used to sell papers at the Trudeau cottages and tried to hold his breath while he made the eight transactions usual in each. He had lived in Saranac all his life and he knew what happened to people who caught the disease.

The more they knew, the more they feared it. John Galbraith, in his book *Playing the Lone Game of Consumption*, quotes a doctor who contracted the disease somewhere about 1916. "To think," said the doctor, "that *I* could get it! Why, it was the one thing I always fled from. If I suspected a patient of having it, I never went to see him twice. I shipped him off to Colorado or Saranac first thing."

The Trudeau Institute had difficulty for a time attracting enough nurses for their patients, for student nurses knew all too well how many of their clan contracted the disease while nursing terminal cases. In 1924 there were well over 800 doctors, medical students and nurses lying in bed in Trudeau at the wrong end of the thermometer. Said Dr. Edward R. Baldwin, director of Trudeau in 1925; "Few [nurses] have had any . . . contact with tuberculosis except in terminal stages . . . such contact fills her with dread. This dread is shared too often by her head nurse or the doctors."

Natives of Saranac say that such was the fear in Saranac's heyday that Al Jolson, planning to perform in the Adirondacks, would not do so until he was shown on the map that the theater was 100 miles from the City of the Sick.

Jack Delahart, who worked at Trudeau for many years and whose uncle had the disease early, describes the moment when after a series of routine X-ray checkups, his last came in positive. "I drove home in a daze, my hands holding the wheel carefully at the very bottom so that I would not have to extend my arms and disturb my lung. I don't know what I would have done if I'd had to swing wide. I knew that raising your arms was bad for sick lungs. Everybody knew that."

He bought a thermometer and took his temperature, which

turned out to be 104. It was widely known in Saranac that such a fever occurred in the worst and terminal cases. All the stories he had heard of the ravages of tuberculosis whirled in his head while he stared at the mercury in his shaking hand. At last he remembered that he'd seen nurses shaking the stick down before taking temperatures, and he got up the courage to do it again. This time he found that it was almost normal, and, feeling reprieved from certain death, he went out and drank a lot of whiskey, positive X-ray or no.

Everybody in Saranac knew the tuberculosis symptoms and the current cure hopes. They knew that the folding cardboard sputum cups the patients carried in their pockets were burned nightly in huge incinerators at the sanitariums because they were dangerous. Lab technicians were especially vulnerable to infection and, deeply immersed in their work, had a habit of telling lurid tales of the short futures of the highly contagious "plus fours," a name for those whose sputum samples were so jammed with bacilli they could scarcely be counted.

No wonder the consumptive was often equated with the leper.

Over in Lake Placid the folks were especially anxious to avoid consumptives. There had never been much love lost between the two villages, separated by only nine miles—some say because of the famous football game in which Saranac took Placid 102 to 0, a game forever enshrined in the annals of history by Ripley in his *Believe It or Not*. But this shellacking was as nothing compared to the fear that the brilliant reputation of Saranac as a cure center would in some degree interfere with the rising fame of Placid's vacation facilities.

Blessed with some of the most matchless scenery in the

country, Placid had established a reputation for winter sports and summer recreation which was drawing more and more fashionable people from New York City, where the heat was as yet unrelieved by air-conditioning and the snow only a nuisance. Hay-fever sufferers had discovered that the same fresh air on which Dr. Trudeau had founded his cure was good for their coughing and sneezing, and just about everybody enjoyed boating and fishing for trout on nearby lakes.

But the Lake Placid Club, sheltering the well-heeled visitors, had daily nightmares that the consumptives would somehow puncture the balloon.

The Club was private and could exclude as it chose. Orders went out, and a discreet sign blossomed on the driveways, "No Tuberculars." At Saranac Inn, the other posh vacation resort of the period, the management also worried, for it was especially difficult to spot the ambulatory tuberculars who, on their high-caloric diets, looked the picture of health and had learned to control their coughs.

The whole country feared the consumptives, but in the Adirondack resorts the tuberculosis victims were as welcome as cases of smallpox at the Paris Exposition.

My mother suffered special unhappiness over the signs which sought to exclude her from the Lake Placid Club. She would avert her eyes from the discreet billboard in front as our car rolled up the drive.

"You mustn't pay it any heed," my father said once as she stared resolutely out the other window.

She shook her head and gave him the ghost of a smile, but even my unobservant eye had caught the glint of tears.

II ❧

An hour's exercise was finally allowed my mother, and no trip to Europe, no visit to the Taj Mahal could have filled her with the same sense of anticipation with which she considered the trip to the village now permitted. An hour meant she could take a taxi with her friends—with Mrs. Diat and with Miss Haas, whose brother was a patient at the Santanoni and would also join them. She could go down into the village, which she had seen only as she passed through it sitting beside my father in the Packard what seemed like centuries ago. She had little memory of what she saw then, having looked at it with a shell-shocked, unseeing stare. She remembered it vaguely as drab and uninteresting, but the thought of seeing it now seemed such a marvelous privilege that she could not fall asleep during naptime and feared her fever would rise and it would all be canceled.

For this major event, just the selection of a suitable dress took hours of thought. The coral wool or the turquoise skirt and a blouse? It was March, but the back of the winter is scarcely broken in Saranac in March, so there would also be galoshes and the squirrel coat. And a cloche. She would have to ease the belt of the dress a bit in any case. The interminable hot cocoa and eggnogs had done their work.

For weeks she and Mrs. Diat had been talking of where they would go for her first expedition and had settled on Sullivan's loan library and then, if there was time, Finnegan's Pharmacy. Not really magnificent destinations, but that was of no importance, and when it was finally time and Mr. Haas's fingers fumbled with the catch of the Santanoni door, she could hardly contain herself lest she miss a minute of the glorious sixty allowed.

They settled back in the cold interior of the cab, all talking at once. Mrs. Diat thought that when my mother was allowed more time, they must certainly lunch at the Riverside Inn, and then of course, much later, they would drive to Lake Placid. Dr. Brown would most certainly approve since he was well known to feel that an hour in a car was beneficial, especially if it were driven at twenty or twenty-five miles per hour. Mr. Haas thought that such a trip would most certainly not be far off.

It had been so long that my mother had lain in bed or on a cure chair that she did not trust her knees, but they laughed her out of her nervousness, explaining that her months of bed rest were no more than average when one considered that Dr. Kinghorn had once put a patient to bed for two years. Her friends vied with each other to point out landmarks, for they had been on three-hour exercise for some time; and then it was time to pay off the cab and walk, actually walk, past the library down to the corner, stopping to peer in windows at the little birchbark canoes and leather photo albums stamped with an Indian head that all the stores displayed. Shopping on Fifth Avenue had never been more exciting.

They passed the Berkeley Hotel, staring up at the windows at the patients sipping their drinks and idly watching the street. They walked slowly, like schoolchildren under the eye of a chaperone, for the important thing was not to hurry, even though there was so much to do and so little time, because a healing lung is vulnerable and must be treated with the same care as a carton of fragile eggs.

They linked arms and laughed, whispering about the people they passed. Once they thought they recognized Carl Palmer, the newspaper magnate whose wife lay ill up on Park Avenue, and once they were sure they saw Lila Lee, the movie star, who was taking the cure at the Adirondack Lodge of National Variety Artists. But each time it turned out to be somebody else after all, and that was somehow funny too.

They selected a novel apiece at Sullivan's, and by then there was very little time left for Finnegan's. They debated going into Jacquemore's in the Hotel Berkeley, where everyone said you might meet an actress, for it was owned by William Morris, the famous theatrical agent, but there was no time. They had barely enough minutes left to step inside the door of Finnegan's and sniff the pungent mixture compounded of unidentifiable parts of things like orris root, Pears' soap, chocolate, rubber hot-water bottles, elastic bandages and sweet, stale air. Then Mr. Haas was looking at his watch and announcing sternly that it was time to go back—it wouldn't do to be late the first time.

They followed him obediently out into the street, nearly colliding with a couple of small boys carrying in their arms a load of baby bottles.

"They pay them a nickel apiece to collect them and then they sell them filled with whiskey," whispered Mr. Haas in my mother's ear, settling into the corner of the cab. "All the drugstores sell liquor that way, and so do the barbers."

They went home the long way around, past the post office and A. Fortune & Co., with its window full of furniture and tapestries.

None of them knew that the top floor of the monstrous green building contained the embalming rooms for Fortune's undertaking business.

It was altogether a very exciting day.

The small boys carrying baby bottles whom my mother encountered coming out of the drugstore were part of a world of which my mother was totally innocent. They were small fry in a large set-up of people looking to make a dishonest dollar by getting around the edge of Prohibition. Many of them are now solid citizens still living in Saranac today.

My mother, in her restricted bird's-eye view of Saranac, could not possibly have understood the undercurrents manifested in such innocent-appearing ways on the streets of the village. Her world was bounded by the dicta of the Santanoni, by her preoccupation with her health and by her status as a respectable matron taking the cure. There was no way she could have really known in what kind of a village she was living. She was an exile, like so many others, but to a large segment of the village, Saranac Lake in the twenties was opportunity incarnate.

The biggest industry of the town was undeniably health, but a close second was contraband liquor, and Saranac, only

134 miles from Montreal and a bit more than 300 from New York City, was a convenient stopover for bootleggers replenishing their supplies for sale in the big city. While the patients lay obediently in their cure chairs and turned out the lights early, the town beneath their windows was awash with smuggling deals, border runs for big money and the visits of some upper-echelon gangsters which this kind of set-up attracted.

There were at least a dozen speakeasies in town which operated more or less within the knowledge of the police. The veterans from World War I, many of whom had contracted tuberculosis, were heavy drinkers. There were also seven stills which manufactured hometown spirits for those who did not want to go all the way to Canada to buy. The stills were marvelously and ingeniously hidden; one in particular, which everyone spoke of breathlessly, was located behind a movable fireplace with an elaborate conduit to an old stump outside in the woods for exhausting fumes. Some of the better stills went so far as to reproduce the glass bottoms of Canadian whiskey bottles, and most sold the liquor labeled with good imitations of the most expensive brands.

Nightly, while the patients slept, the supply of genuine Canadian booze in Saranac was replenished by small-time liquor runners who made the trip into Canada, braving the famous Black Horse Brigade, Troop B, established in 1921 to cover the border in pairs on horseback. Souped-up Cadillacs, Packards and Marmons equipped with special springs to enable them to ride inconspicuously with twenty to twenty-five cases as freight on the way back lurked in carefully camouflaged hideaways, waiting for the right signal, often given by a cooperating officer of the law, to sally forth for a night's work.

So much money changed hands every night in Saranac that

men hoisting a few in a speak were complaining that laying off the run to get an occasional night's sleep cost them upward of $100. It was whispered in the town that even the head nun at St. Mary's sanitarium was cooperating a bit—all, of course, for the sake of the patients' welfare. It was said she gave one of the local bootleggers alcohol which he doctored up for resale. Eugene Keough, who still runs one of the town's three undertaking establishments, said that once when he was sent on an errand by his boss, he stubbed his toe and $325,000 in cash, all goldback $20 bills, spilled out of the grocery sack he was carrying. Down at the St. Regis Hotel one of the entrepreneurs got to thinking he would like to own a place like that and pulled out a roll of $100,000 to prove he meant business. Mr. Morgan, the owner, turned him down. It is not recorded why.

All during Prohibition the Black Horse Brigade relied on horses to navigate those snow-choked roads crossing the Canadian border from upper New York State. The captain, C. J. Broadfield, had a Ford, and the troopers divided four Harley-Davison motorcycles amongst them, but chiefly the law enforcers were mounted. Very shortly, however, this unequal balance of equipment between law and lawbreakers was rectified, for the troopers captured a good share of the cars making the run and could thereafter more than keep up. They were diligent in their pursuit of the booze runners, chasing them in their own cars, attired in uniforms topped with black Stetsons reminiscent of Nelson Eddy's early costumes, implementing President Coolidge's orders twenty-four hours a day. They carried Colt. 45's and Winchester .30-.30's, and their pay was a munificent $900 a year. They were based in Malone, and their whereabouts at any given time was a matter of intense interest.

They were largely unloved. Prohibition was not a popular

amendment, and most people, especially in the frozen north country, considered it their inalienable right to be able to swallow a tot of liquor of an evening to keep out the cold. Canadian stool pigeons sometimes squealed on the men making the run, but in Saranac the sympathy was with the wets. They were largely local men who had started small with secondhand cars, fixed them up with armor plating and smoke-screen devices and built up a little nest egg. You could buy a case of Canadian ale for $240 in a Canadian border town. Just across the line, it instantly became worth $700.

One among many was Kootchie Hale, a Saranac citizen who, like so many, got into the business because he needed the money. He made a fortune and lost it. Like most local men, he specialized in wines and beers. Sometimes he would drive a load all the way into New York City, where his connections put him up at the best hotels, usually in a suite. He had two sets of plates for his souped-up car and would register it with one set going into Canada and then, before coming home, put on the others.

Kootchie's wife was reluctant to have him involved in booze running, but the first time he tried it and slipped through the roving patrol undetected, he went down to Jack Moore's, one of Saranac's finest stores, and bought her a pink coat with a white lining. He paid $35 for it, a lot of money in those days, and she was, in Kootchie's own words, tickled pink.

Still she was nervous and kept at him to quit, but it was such easy money. They argued about it, and he promised after a while he would retire, pointing out that it was risky but lucrative.

It was risky, all right, but the money was really too good. The men drove at night without lights and came across the border at varying places, preceded by a pilot to divert the suspicions of the police, should they be around. The pilot's job was to allow himself to be searched while back a ways at the crossroads, the real load was waiting for the signal. If the pilot didn't come back in twenty minutes, the driver with the whiskey would take another road.

Kootchie remembers a night which many of his friends could probably match, but which lingers in his mind particularly because his baby girl had just been born.

He was feeling good, driving along with a full load, singing to himself and thinking life was treating him pretty well. And then all of a sudden it was as if he were on stage—everything was lit up bright as day, says Kootchie—and ahead were six or seven formerly bootleggers' souped-up cars in the possession of the police.

He'd been caught once and it would have meant two years in prison this time, so he slowed down to put them off the scent, double-clutched the Packard and put the accelerator to the floor. He went right by them, and a trooper dropped to one knee as he passed and put two bullets through the front door. Kootchie kept going. The boys in the black hats got in the cars and gave chase, and after a while they were gaining on him, so he got out on the running board, twisted the wheel of the Packard for a sharp turn off the road and jumped. The Packard careened across a field, but he hid in the woods and hitched a ride home with a fruit peddler.

The pilot, released as they nearly always were because they were clean, sought out Kootchie the next night at home. He went in to look at the new baby and pay his respects to Mrs. Hale and then, in spite of frantic signals from Kootchie, he asked her if she knew she was almost a widow the night before. She was still in bed after the birth of the baby, and she raised herself up on one elbow and looked her husband in the eye and said, "Choose, Kootchie, booze running or me."

Kootchie was in a bad spot and he glared at the pilot, a big, good-looking blond kid not overburdened with sensitivity. He tried to soothe his wife, but there was no calming her down till the pilot, with a stroke of genius, solved the whole situation by telling Mrs. Hale that booze running was indeed too dangerous for her husband and in the future he would drive the Packard and let Kootchie run interference.

What he didn't tell her was that the troopers hated the pilots because they were hard to get the goods on and if they caught one through a tip, they would put him away for far longer than the actual driver. Mrs. Hale did not know this and was satisfied. Kootchie continued to make the border run, on and off in various capacities, for fourteen years.

He got very good at it, as did all those who survived, eluding the troopers by throwing out roofing nails or broken glass to blow their tires, but always worried that a shot would get the gas tank and send him sky-high. He finally had a blacksmith put a shield around the tank, and then he breathed easier. Still and all, he had to abandon at least a car a year, and many nights he had to sleep in the current automobile with its incriminating load.

It was a difficult life, but there are memories. Once he delivered six cases of 1911 Cliquot Club champagne to Paul Smith's when Coolidge's summer White House was there and the troopers were as thick as flies on the road. Later he drank champagne himself at the Hotsy Totsy Club in New York, $22 a bottle for the same stuff he was importing, and Lillian and Dorothy Gish were seated at the next table. The Hotsy Totsy Club was owned by Legs Diamond, a notorious bootlegger known as the "Clay Pigeon" because he had taken so many bullets in his body and survived. Kootchie had come a long way from the first Peerless he bought for the business secondhand for $600.

But in the end it all faded away.

There were many like Kootchie in Saranac, according to all accounts, and sometimes the police could be bought off for a dollar a case. There was one who raced his motorcycle to signal the all-clear for the cars hidden in the warehouse down by the depot. The town fathers themselves were no bluenoses, and Kootchie, who operated a taxi as a front, says he remembers once bringing home the town judge, the town clerk, the mayor and the district attorney, all so inebriated they couldn't manage to step up on the running board. Down at the Pines Club things were more respectable, but they were drinking the wine supplied by Kootchie.

Saranac Lake, almost as north and east as you can get, had in the twenties a fundamental resemblance to the Western frontier towns of an earlier age. Just three or four decades removed from a mountain trading post, long isolated from civilization in its frozen setting unblemished by roads, it had all the attributes of a gold prospector who, after years of grubstaking, has come into the money. From a village consisting of a sawmill, a small hotel for guides and lumbermen, a country store, a schoolhouse and a dozen guides' homes, it had suddenly blossomed into a town full of people who could buy expensive furs, jewels, champagne and baskets of hothouse fruit and flowers. Its streets, which had recently known only the boots of trappers and guides, were now filled with celebrities, monied socialites—and some of the most successful and innovative crooks and gangsters in the business.

The roaring twenties roared particularly in Saranac. A man was shot standing on the porch of the Riverside Inn in this period, and nobody ever found out who did it or why. The place was full of small feuds among the underworld, full of liquored-up people with guns. Some of them had real flair.

Like the ones who robbed Edelberg's fur shop next door to the Pontiac Theatre just as the lines for the show were being let in.

Morris and Sam Edelberg were two brothers who had followed the money to Saranac and were in competition with each other for the patronage of the women who could afford mink, sable and beaver. Sam had a slightly better clientele, it was generally acknowledged, and it was his shop the crooks hit. While a streetful of waiting theater patrons looked on, they propped the door to his shop wide open and loaded the contents of the store into a waiting truck on Broadway.

An idle bystander inquired what was going on. The two cool robbers replied that Sam wanted the furs all sent back to New York for glazing. The truck was blocking traffic on narrow Broadway, and the cop on the corner came over to see what was going on. He ended up helping to load the furs.

They got away clean. That's the kind of town Saranac was.

❧ 12

My mother's fever chart showed no climb after her first exercise, and Dr. Brown was well pleased. Little by little, he allowed her five more minutes a day, a step or two up and down was added to her privileges, and at last she was part of the group that could rent a Chris-Craft at Pleasant Bay boathouse, take a picnic lunch and spend as much as three hours away from the Santanoni.

It was late summer by now and the sun on the mountainside late in the evening was something that almost made it worth while to have to lie on the porch and watch. There were parties, picnics, outings of all kinds—but not every day, only occasionally, for the watchword was rest and everything else had to be fitted in around this. It was summer, but the nights were already cool and the men wore white flannels which were not a bit too warm and the women needed sweaters.

It was harder to drink the milk and the eggnog when what one wanted was lemonade in a tall glass with tinkling ice, but nothing had really changed, only the leash had been let out a little longer. There were still the constant card games and discussions about the next entertainment, and always the feeling, when the lights were coming on and the mountains turning purple in the shadows, that real life was going on somewhere else and this was only a kind of hiatus, a time out in their existence which would be picked up like a dropped stitch later.

There was one sadness. Mr. Haas was once more confined to his bed with fever. He was very brave about it and said he was sure he would be right as rain in no time, but when he didn't think anyone was watching, his eyes looked very discouraged. He was forbidden to read or talk during naptime and was receiving no visitors except his sister. In the dining room and over the bridge table, the ambulatory patients looked solemn when his name was mentioned. In Saranac the retrogression of any patient was a sadness to all. It was a reminder to each that next time it might be he.

It was in this late summer that the first death occurred since my mother's arrival at the Santanoni. It was not anyone she knew—it was someone who had never, as long as she had been there, emerged from a top-floor suite with two private nurses—but it nevertheless cast her into a deep funk. My father, arriving for the weekend full of joviality at her recent progress, stared in consternation at her face.

"But you didn't know him," he protested. "He was just a name to you."

"It doesn't matter," said my mother. "I knew him. He was me, he was all of us."

She was staring at the mountains as if she had never seen them before.

"Was it very sudden?" inquired my father, at last able to see that she must talk about it.

She told him all she knew—the clip-clop of the horses' feet bringing the ice to weight his chest in a last-ditch hope of quieting the hemorrhage, the doctors coming and going, and the quick grapevine that told them when at last it was too late. When she had finished, she was crying, for a man she had never met.

Or maybe for all of them in the big pseudo-Tudor sanitarium on the hill.

"You're better, Bess," said my father, putting his arms around her.

She went on looking at the mountains.

They died in the Santanoni as they died in Ray Brook, though not so often, so that it was more of an unaccustomed trauma. And it was very difficult for the undertakers in the Santanoni, for the stairs were too narrow for a stretcher and the elevator was very cramped. Eugene Keough, of the Keough Funeral Home, says that many a time he got into the Santanoni elevator with a corpse cradled like a baby in his arms, for there was no other way to remove the body. He would sit on the elevator stool with the remains in his arms, waiting patiently for the elevator to make its majestic way down.

Eugene is one of the few people who lived in Saranac for years and never had tuberculosis. His boss was Henry Conley, who built the funeral parlor in 1909. Conley came up from Brooklyn with his father, who had the disease, and an uncle and an aunt, and at Thendara his father hemorrhaged so badly they had to take him off the train. He cured at 33 Franklin Avenue, Mrs. McCabe's, and recovered.

Conley always wore gloves when he prepared the remains, for he knew first hand what it was like to have tuberculosis. The general feeling in Albany at the time was that corpses were likely to be extremely contagious—"plus fours," as the labs referred to them. But Eugene said that wearing gloves in his work was like taking a bath with your shoes on, and he wouldn't put them on. He says he buried hundreds and thousands of "plus fours," but remained healthy. Dr. Hayes, one of the prominent specialists, who lived next door, couldn't believe Eugene's remarkable luck. The bodies, of course, were not breathing, but the blood, as Eugene explains it, is a kind of cesspool for everything after death, and he was drawing it off to make room for formaldehyde. Dr. Hayes considered writing a paper on Eugene's splendid health under the circumstances, but never got around to it. He concluded that Eugene had developed an immunity.

Saranac was full of patients from South America, most of them young and rich. Many didn't arrive until the disease was far advanced, and not a few died quite early after arrival. South American families were always especially anxious to bury the bodies at home, but the law in some of the countries was a problem because it forbade bringing in the body of a tubercular victim until fifteen years had passed.

Eugene especially remembers the death of a young man from Colombia whose family was extremely wealthy and unusually anxious to bury their son at home in the family plot.

The embassy in Washington was approached with a petition to relax the rules, but was adamant. Dr. Francis Trudeau, senior, a man of strong principles and the doctor in the case, refused to cooperate in filling out the death certificate. "To him," says Eugene, "there was white and black, and there was no changing that." Cause of death was duly listed as tuberculosis.

But the deceased's family was determined to bring their son home, no matter how long it took. Accordingly, the Keough Funeral Home put the young man's body in a crypt, and fifteen years later to the day, a cable arrived requesting that, now that the time period had elapsed, the bones of the young man be sent home. Keough cabled back that they were sending vault and all because the body was probably in good shape. The family found this hard to believe, but approved shipment.

Vault and body waited several days on the wharf for a banana boat going back home, while the family in Colombia nervously awaited its arrival. Two days after the boat pulled into harbor, the Keough Funeral Home received an excited phone call. Relatives had opened the vault with a blowtorch and discovered that, except for a little dehydration and what the funeral people refer to as a tan, their son looked better than when he was sick. They wanted Keough to know that they had called in all the family, fifteen years later, and were holding a second funeral.

Many died, obscure and famous, and one of the most notorious victims of the disease was Legs Diamond's brother, Eddie. During the long, unsuccessful cure, it is said that Eddie's bodyguard had had to lie in a cure chair next to Eddie, bound by the restrictions imposed on his charge.

Legs paid his brother quite a few calls during the period when Eddie lay vainly attempting to recover his health in Saranac; he was always careful to keep a low profile, for he was a much wanted man, not only by the police but by Dutch Schultz, into whose territory he was muscling. He assumed various costumes to throw his pursuers off the scene—once he wore a nun's habit—but the night he came to arrange for Eddie's funeral is the one Saranac still remembers.

Eugene Keough was at the time a young assistant in the business which he was later to buy. It was he who answered the doorbell to let in a woman in a large hat accompanied by a man asking for Mr. Conley.

Eugene says he was caught by the odd appearance of the woman, particularly her legs, which were sturdy and hairy. He seemed unable to remove his eyes from her, a fact which did not escape the attention of her escort. After leading them to Conley's office, Eugene could not help but pause briefly in the doorway for one last look.

"Who are you?" growled the man.

Conley explained that this was his assistant.

The man continued to glare, studying Eugene with a pair of hard eyes flat with suspicion.

"Beat it, kid," he said finally.

When the pair had taken their departure, Conley called Eugene to his office. Without a word he indicated the clay figures of the three monkeys—blind, deaf and dumb to evil— which sat on his desk.

Then he said they had a big job for which they would be well paid. They would be preparing the body, though the funeral would be in New York City. He said he himself would drive the hearse to the train and that Eugene would drive the bereaved in the black Packard. He would accompany the body all the way to Tupper Lake, the junction where Eugene would pick him up after delivering his passengers to the train.

Eugene was ready at the appointed time, opening the Packard door with downcast eyes to the pair he had seen in the office earlier. All the way to Tupper Lake behind the wheel of the Packard he could see in the rear-view mirror the odd pair staring silently ahead of them. Stuck in the belt of the man were what could only be two pistols.

Connections were smoothly made, and Eugene picked up his boss, who then confided to him that his passengers had been Legs Diamond dressed as a woman, accompanied by his bodyguard. But Legs never made his brother's funeral. He got off the train at Albany on a tip that there would be an ambush, and he was shot down on Dove Street in a dingy roominghouse. Eddie Diamond's wife, a pretty blonde and the mother of two children, didn't live much longer. The underworld decided she knew more than they cared her to and rubbed her out.

13 ❧

The following year my mother at last had improved enough so that my father felt it worth while to rent a house in Saranac for the summer so that we could be near her. In my mind's eye I walk up the front walk of that brown-shingled house on Park Avenue, see the screened sleeping porch which was so large it turned the corner, and look out a window bordering on the mountains. But I do not know where it was. My brother, in a rare moment of confidence, told me that it belonged to Irene Castle, but this is not so, for I have it on good authority that Irene Castle passed only momentarily through Saranac to call on her agent, William Morris, in his beautiful Camp Intermission and never had a house. Everyone who would remember now is gone. I have driven the block where I thought it was repeatedly, but it is not there. Perhaps it burned, as so many of the Adirondack houses did, from an overheated furnace or sometimes, it is whispered, for the insurance.

At any rate, the Packard rolled majestically up to the door of this house the summer I was five, bringing me, my brother, the three dogs, my nurse, Anna, and, though I cannot remember her, a cook. The car turned up the driveway and disgorged us from its capacious interior to spend three months, more or less, in the shadow of Mount Pisgah. I vaguely remember toiling up the sides of this gently sloping, tree-covered mountain in my brother's wake and bringing back samples of foliage and pieces of fungus on which we always drew domestic scenes which included the dogs and, without fail, a brightly shining sun in the upper right-hand corner.

I can walk through that house now in my memory, but I do not find my mother in it. She kept mostly to her apartment in the Santanoni, observing the nap periods, keeping her excursions with us to the prescribed limits, leaving us to the servants to manage during the week. We seldom went to see her, for it was not thought wise for us to enter the Santanoni any more than necessary. Our meetings with our mother took place in the sharp mountain air over picnic baskets, in boats, across dining-room tables in resorts that did not cater to consumptives.

There were many families like ours, I think, in Saranac, but we did not know them. We did not go to the Baldwin School in the winter, where so many of the children of patients made their friends. It was run by the wife of a patient, a Wellesley graduate who turned to the idea of the school as a desperate last-ditch way to support her ill husband. Because she was a sister-in-law of Dr. Edward Baldwin, one of the great tuberculosis specialists, her connections were good, and the school was a success. But we did not attend, nor were we allowed to take the very large automobile with the folding seats which lumbered as a shuttle between Broadway and Trudeau, on which so many of the neighborhood children rode during rest hours when the patients would all be safely in bed.

Thus, we two were thrown back on our own resources, or, rather, my brother was reduced to playing with me. I suppose it must have been lonely for him, but I wasn't aware of it then as he taught me to identify birds' eggs and impressed me to help with the projects suggested in Ernest Thompson Seton's nature books. We might have been on an island, for even our help was not local, so that we heard none of the delicious behind-the-scenes gossip to which other children were privy in their kitchens—what celebrity was visiting this week next door, and how poor, ill Mr. So-and-so was coming along.

Most difficult of all, of course, was the role of my father, who came only on weekends. His life during the week went on as usual in the lumberyard and in the house on Maple Street. He was in great demand as an extra man, but there were many nights when he must have dined alone. It would make a better story to say he fell in love and was torn between his duty to his invalid wife and his mistress, but it was not that way. Except for the very early years, my parents' life was always a series of separations, of fragmented family life, of long-distance phone calls and of leaving children with servants. In our absence the same town of which we were so much a part understood this and enfolded my father in its social life.

In the Santanoni the cheerful cousining of Trudeau, the gallows humor and the slang which referred to a hemorrhage as a ruby and a consumptive as a lunger were muted. Still, though the Santanoni was self-contained, the residents were subject to the same occupational hazards as the rest of the patients in Saranac. They, too, developed intensive relationships, close friendships founded on the similarities of their highly distinctive lives.

They spent long hours comparing temperatures and conducting introspective dialogues. The long, long progress of the disease and the irksome restrictions bound them together in a life where preoccupation with self blurred into an insidious acceptance of an existence which only another patient could understand. Little by little, they became like the passengers on a long ocean voyage, suspended between real worlds with fellow passengers whose interests and problems were identical. What was in Trudeau and Ray Brook a simple, blithe and easygoing, often sexual relationship flowered in the more rarefied atmosphere of the Santanoni in somewhat subtler forms of flirtation, deep affinity and, inevitably, sometimes divorce.

I cannot say that my mother did or did not form the kind of liaison which blossomed all around her, but I believe she did not. If she had, I think some hint of it would have drifted down to me over the years.

Still, I imagine that my father was aware of all this, and I think the house on Park Avenue was part of my father's effort to bring some sort of normal family life to her and, as he kept making me implore the Lord, to "bring the whole family together again."

In the houses on Park Avenue and in the Glenwood estates were many other families making the same kind of effort to keep together, some unsuccessfully. It would be interesting to know what the divorce rate of Saranac was in the twenties, when legal separation was considered somewhat unusual elsewhere. The constant presence of money from the big cities and foreign capitals made the morals of Saranac immeasurably freer than in most small villages. In the upper social strata, affairs and divorces were certainly more common than in the economically pressed circles, where the style was downright desertion and abandonment.

But in our new life only yards from the famous gates of Trudeau Institute, we did not know any of this. We simply lived for the weekend—and for those occasional days in the middle of the week which my father, working in a family business, could steal. He would come into the house smelling familiarly of tobacco and tweed, and the whole day would come suddenly alive. With my mother beside him on the front seat, we would drive to the nearby resorts—to Lake Clear Inn, then popular with the families of patients who worried about bringing young children to Saranac itself, to the Lake Placid Club or to the old Saranac Inn.

I learned to swim in Lake Clear while my parents sorted their lives out in the shade of the dock. I learned to sit up straight and hold my fork correctly while they exchanged news of the week's events. I seemed always to be seated across from them in some resort whose proprietors did not know my mother was ill, eating my way through a three-course dinner as the light faded.

Those summers that we rented the Saranac house blur into each other like the colors of a child's water-paint drawing, but in my memory I am always on my best behavior, seated across from my mother, who is now round-faced and healthy-looking and engaged in trying to hide the food under knife and fork. It did not distress me to hear that she was not hungry. It was a fact that piqued my interest, and I remember leaning forward eagerly to hear the answer when my brother asked her if she skipped one meal, would she not be ravenous for the next.

"No," she said simply, rearranging the food on her plate.

All the resorts refused entry to known tuberculars, and of all of them, the Lake Placid Club was the most strict. Dr. Brown did not encourage coughing, but as we rounded Mirror Lake on the approach to the Club, we nearly always stopped to see if my mother needed to cough before entering. The management knew that cough.

There were many gentle outings, often with Miss Haas and her brother, now once again improved. Those two made my mother laugh, but I wished there had been other children for me to talk to as we took the leisurely rides among the mountains or the excursion sightseeing launch from Lake Flower up through the Saranac River to the marina on Lower Saranac Lake. The lake was full of islands and very beautiful, and it was a favorite weekend amusement for us.

The trip was captained by Harold Thomas, who enlivened it with outrageous tales of what the famous had done in the area. I don't remember this, but Alice Wareham, daughter of John Ridenour who owned the *Enterprise*, says Captain Thomas delighted in pointing out, as we passed, a particular big rock which, he said, was the very same from which "the sisters Irene and Verne Castle did their famous jump." Since nearly all of Captain Thomas' passengers knew, as he didn't, that Vernon was Irene's husband, there was much merriment and suppressed giggles at his expense.

It was an innocent life in which we children thought, and our parents pretended, that we were not really very different from other families elsewhere, other summer vacationers, hoisting our picnic basket in the brief July sun, settling ourselves into the pleasure launches. It was a summer idyll with a fatal flaw, but, like an internal wound, it was not visible to the naked eye, and we never spoke of it. With the adaptability of children, we assumed that what happened to us was much like what happened to most. There was no sense of tragedy; you cannot live for long periods fearing the worst. We were simply a family with special rules which would, no doubt, be relaxed next month, next year, soon.

Our parents did their best to foster this unspoken conspiracy to deny that we were different. In a way which could never be managed today in the small houses in which we live so closely, they kept us ignorant of how things really were. *Pas devant les enfants*—and the servants, who must have known more about my mother's condition and our future, honored the plot to keep us in the dark. We were not to worry; grown-ups would manage things. "Mrs. C. was sick and has gone away for a while," a friend of mine at home was told. "When she comes home, she will be all better."

At all costs they preserved the fiction that nothing bad could happen, that life would unravel forever as untroubled and bland as vanilla pudding.

In my parents' circles this was simply the way things were. The real decisions and announcements were made behind closed doors, in halls outside our rooms when we were in bed. I cannot remember anyone ever telling me that my mother was better or worse, that the fever charts had developed alarming peaks or that, alternately, she had gained a few pounds. Disease was outside the province of childhood, and tuberculosis, except for its attendant need for scrubbing our hands and keeping our distance, was not much discussed in our presence.

Naturally, we children became extremely adept at picking up what we were not supposed to, though in those early years I was much too young to notice. But my brother, four years older, saw to it that my state of grace was brief. He was a surrogate parent to me, stern and cold. He knew things I did not, and it was from him that I learned the basic unpleasant facts of life, such as that there was no Santa Claus. "Mother and Dad do it all," he told me quite gratuitously one day, lying on his stomach in the library. I hadn't asked, but I knew there was no appeal from what he said. He was privy to information I was not.

It was also he who told me that Mother had had a relapse.

14 ✤

"It never occurred to me before I was married," said my father, kicking the logs in the fireplace so that they settled into a bright, steady blaze, "that money was for things like dentists or doctors or insurance or taxes. I thought it was for the theater and trips to Nassau. Or a new car or a fur coat."

I knew even then he wasn't complaining. He was remarking on a fact.

He straightened up and replaced the screen over the fireplace. "And I thought your mother would always be right there, sitting in the chair opposite me at dinner, beside me in the car, in the fur coat."

He looked at me absently, only vaguely aware of his audience.

"I suppose in some ways it's even harder on you," he said, but I could see he didn't think so.

"I guess you miss her, too."

I nodded dumbly.

It was one of his few unguarded moments. I had a mother and yet I didn't, and I learned almost nothing of her from him. It was only years later, kneeling in front of an old doll's trunk that belonged to her when she was a girl, that I began to understand what it must have been like in those years away from us. Children are slow to imagine what happens to grown-ups, especially what happens in other places. Only now that I am older than she ever lived to be can I peel away the years from my image of her to find the young woman peering so seriously out at me from under her wedding veil, unaware what lies ahead of her.

It is a search, a puzzle with many pieces missing, but in this trunk are leftover parts of her life. There, among old love letters and childish scrawls from me written home from camp, I found her medical diaries.

Small and brown, with only her name and the dates on the covers, in her own handwriting, they are stacked neatly in one corner. They might be composition books for a child just learning to write, but once opened, they condense the history of her life in Saranac. One is missing—they are clearly numbered in the upper right-hand corner of the cover as if she knew there would be more than one from the beginning. Each is a year of her life, distilled into temperature readings, symptoms, penciled notes of whom she saw, what she did, how she felt, all coordinated to the fever chart for the doctor's guidance.

Each begins with instructions. Keep the thermometer in your mouth never less than five minutes; in cold weather or out of doors, the mouth should be closed on the stick for fifteen minutes. When the temperature reaches 100 and stays there two hours, go to bed.

There are places to note symptoms—faintness, dizziness, insomnia, nervousness, indigestion. Neat boxes await notations about decrease or increase of cough, expectoration (increased? decreased? blood?), a shortness of breath. Hours in bed are to be recorded, the amount of exercise allowed and appetite, weight and pulse rate.

What kind of diary is this for a woman barely out of her twenties?

But it is the one she had to keep, and, holding it in my hand, I am struck once again by how things outlast people, remaining to make a chain of continuity when the person who owned them is gone. My mother, so reticent about her disease, has in the end told me everything.

I turn the pages with their neat notations, and such is the power of the earlier fear that, when I have finished, I am ashamed but I feel I must wash my hands.

She kept the books religiously at first—pulse, insomnia, everything. But as the weeks went by she obviously wearied of this and reduced the medical notations to a simple fever chart accompanied by marginal scribbles telling who came to visit, how she felt and what kind of weather lay outside her window.

Page after page of the temperature readings look remarkably similar, a graphic reflection of a long-drawn-out illness. The three daily readings connected by lines make a series of little drunken tents, like the border of an Oriental rug whose maker knows the gods are jealous of perfection and purposely weaves the pattern awry.

But then suddenly, on one of the pages, a huge crazy line

rises straight up into the margin where there is no place even to record such a temperature. The picture of her relapse is drawn there in faded brown ink, as if some malevolent spirit had jiggled her hand. One hundred four, point six.

There are no clues in the little brown book to what caused this crazy jagged line in the rug pattern on an otherwise uneventful day in mid-October. A ride, as usual, says the chart, dressed for two hours, a quiet day.

But the rest of October's and November's pages are blank. The lines of communication are down, snapped like a telephone line, until the notations resume once more on the 21st of December, the little tents again well-behaved miniatures below the normal line. Dr. Brown came in on that December evening, and she received her last hypo. There are no notes of visitors or rides or movies. Her weight had come up to 124. December 25 is only another little unremarked tent on the chart.

Seven weeks out of her life are missing.

It happened so often to so many patients in the twenties— the cruel drop back into the pit after the slow climb to normality. For TB was a disease which, like the performing circus tiger, appears to be tamed but awaits only an opportunity to revert to savagery. Relapse was the hallmark of the disease, even if you followed the doctor's orders conscientiously. Fear of just what happened to my mother was what kept every patient lying in a sleeping porch from cheating on medical orders. They knew how easy it was to think that the worst was behind and then find you had slipped back into the original nightmare.

Nobody discussed those weeks in my hearing. But in her penciled note in the margin, it is all encapsuled.

"Les semaines de l'enfer," she wrote in the little brown book.

My father, as usual, kept the knowledge from us. He took the train back up to Saranac by way of Utica, the roads over the back way being uncertain if not impassable, and was gone several nights. Anna professed ignorance of why he had returned so soon to Saranac, but my brother had heard the talk in the kitchen.

My mother's trouble seeped into my consciousness the same way the Depression was later to do, as a *fait accompli,* an important event which happened offstage and which everyone else had always known.

It did not even loom large in my life. I had started kindergarten that fall and was allowed to go by myself to the school two blocks through alleys behind our house. I lay awake nightly, but not because my mother was desperately ill. I was terrified that I would be late for school, sure that only a perfect punctuality record stood between me and the beating with a rubber hose which was whispered of in the hall. I was afraid to close my eyes for fear the opening bell would clang without me. I knew so little about my mother and she about me. My mother had always been sick. She was a little sicker. She would get better.

But I remember the aunties and courtesy aunties clustering round, petting me as if I had suddenly become very fragile.

"I'm going to steal the child and take her to Utica today," says one to Anna, viewing with a slight moue the Dutch bob my father's barber had wrought. "She needs a proper haircut and perhaps a nice dress."

What my father thought is impossible to know. He returned from Saranac, took supper with us and talked of other things. Mother had sent her love. We were to write, both of us. And how was school?

"For other diseases, we may buy a cure," wrote a patient in Trudeau in 1906. "Not consumptives. Patience and perseverance in leading a hygienic life are the only specifics for it."

My mother's setback was part of the pattern, a personal tragedy of which the doctors had seen hundreds. Many, especially those on whom the financial difficulties of curing fell hardest, began to feel better after a few months, cut loose and went home, only to have the fever return and the cough become once more racking and blood-stained. Many tried to do too much, too early, and paid for it.

A combination of chest thumping, X-rays and temperature charts gave the doctors a reasonable idea of the progress of the disease, but it was only partly accurate. At best they were blundering along in half-knowledge. A cavity heals, another could well open. There was no guarantee that what had happened before could not happen again. The disease might be only quiescent. Well aware of this, many who returned to an active life with what they prayed were inactive cases hedged their bets by trying to keep doing what they had done in Saranac.

They changed their occupations from indoor to outdoor, hoping to shift the odds in their favor. The financially pressed left factory or clerical work to drive cabs or sell papers. The affluent threw over lucrative administrative positions in industry to buy rambling hotels in out-of-the-way vacation spots so that they could still spend eight hours in the fresh air.

Knowledge of this did not much cheer my mother, lying again in bed, the parties and excursions going on without her. She lay watching from the confines of her porch a third

Saranac winter gather force, and now it was doubly hard, for she was already beginning to feel better. She stared at the snowflakes swirling in eddies before a gusty north wind and wondered bleakly if she would still be lying there when they were once more beginning to melt.

Soon after Christmas she was once more allowed visitors, and on the 4th of January my father came again. She had gained six pounds, he told us when he came home, but his face looked so closed that even I, obsessed with my punctuality record, noticed it.

It was her friends at the Santanoni, he told me later, who pulled her back up into the world. They would not allow her to despair. They were like a club, a very private and exclusive club, the initiation into which might well be a hemorrhage, and she was one of their own. As soon as Dr. Brown would allow it, they came in relays, telling her stories of how they themselves had experienced just such an unhappy episode and had promptly recovered. They reminded her of how Mr. Haas had been put to bed and was now again going about everywhere. They reminded her that her temperature was once more below the danger line, they had already heard, and predicted she would be dining with them again before the next premiere at the Pontiac.

She told them what she could not tell my father, that she was frightened that she had galloping consumption and would fade quite away shortly, and they said in chorus that it couldn't be true because she was already almost three years into the cure and still alive. No consolation from the outside world could possibly have cheered her as they did, for they spoke to her from shared knowledge of how it was. She was traveling territory familiar to all of them.

When they saw that she felt better, they began at once to

plan one of their eternal expeditions to Placid. For next month, they said, because by then they were sure she would be able to go. Did she think it should be for lunch or dinner? To the Club, perhaps, or would she prefer the Riverside Inn?

Some consumptives did indeed die very quickly, without warning, in Saranac. Almost overnight, it seemed, they lost their hold on the world and slipped away. It was a special form of tuberculosis, known in the early part of this century as galloping consumption, and its very name made every patient shiver. Victims of galloping consumption died without leaving their beds, but usually the cure, or sometimes the long, unsuccessful battle, took place over a matter of years. A long, long convalescence marked with ups and downs was the rule, and it is no wonder friends made along the way were closer than blood. Becalmed on a raft together, with no way to summon help, the passengers could hardly remain casual acquaintances.

At the Santanoni this was truer than anywhere else, for a common economic background brought together people with similar tastes, and their small, enclosed world with its strange rules bound them closer at once. They were like members of a large family, snowbound together in one eternal house party.

A large family whose coat-of-arms might well have been crossed thermometers, with a pair of galoshes rampant, and the motto above emblazoned in red, *"Carpe Diem."*

My mother's large extended family would not allow her to despair.

15 ❧

"Do you remember what it was like when Mother was so sick?" I ask my brother. "Did she speak of it afterward to you?"

He only shakes his head.

I wear her engagement ring. Her wedding dress with a tiny wine stain on it still hangs in my closet, the little diamond pendant my father gave her when they married is in my jewelry box, but these things are almost all I have of her. I can scarcely remember anything of consequence she said to me. Perhaps she meant to keep it that way in the little bit of time we were together.

She was fond of a special kind of Dutch coffee candy and of

jujubes. She extravagantly admired Sherlock Holmes. Leslie Howard was her idol—she saw every one of his plays and movies. She had been through everything of Dickens' more than once. Because of her I read Dickens far too early and was put off for years. These are the things about her stored in the attic of my mind, and they are almost all I have to take out when I think of her.

"Why won't Ed tell me what he remembers about her?" I ask his wife.

"She was very special to him," she replies in the same voice she used to use when I was too young to go to their parties.

"But she was my mother, too," I cry, resisting an impulse to stamp my foot.

But she only shrugs.

All right. I piece her together without their help—from the diaries, the letters and the things my father, at last breaking the code which forbade discussing personal things with one's children, told me. And from the contents of the Victorian doll's trunk lined with rose-decorated wallpaper and a picture of a Gibson Girl wearing a big hat.

"My train was late," she writes to my father, "and there was no one in the station last night. So I thought I'd take a peek in the club and call up my house or perhaps find Emily and Bill to see me home. I was really looking for you, but as I cautiously applied my eye to the window at the club, I saw only Newell and Antoinette inside. So I tiptoed down the walk again and made for the streetcar. I want to see you so much."

The letter is written on Waldorf-Astoria paper—she must have been on a visit or perhaps it was the year she was at finishing school in New York—and it is hard for me to believe my eyes. My controlled and elegant mother tiptoeing up the walk to peek through the windows of a men's club, looking for a man to whom she is not even yet engaged. I cannot reconcile it with my images of her walking so carefully down the walk beside me, stopping to rest a moment before climbing the running board of the LaSalle.

"Jamais je ne t'oublerai pas," says the little poem in her handwriting that somehow has been left behind for me to see. I think she is the author from the way a word here and there is changed. Then there were moments when she cared deeply, loved achingly and let somebody, perhaps my father, know it. "I am *sick* to see you," she writes, and this time it is certainly to my father.

It is hard to make her into the same woman who lay in the big brass bed talking with me one day when I was perhaps seven.

I was inquiring about sex.

"How can you tell," I was asking her, remembering to keep the required safe distance across the room between us, "whether it's a boy or a girl if they're a baby and not wearing blue or pink?"

I can still hear the stillness in the room.

"Don't you know?" she said at last.

I shook my head, but the conversation died there. I learned in the usual way of my generation the next summer at camp.

I do not bring her to task for this. She searched in her mind for a way to tell me—I could see that. It was just not the kind of conversation in which she felt at home.

"I try to remember a moment when I talked to my mother and we said something, but I can't," says a friend of mine.

It was simply the way it was in that time.

She was an anti-suffragist. I know it because I discovered this in one of her letters.

"The suffrage meetings are the best thing I've done, very amusing," she writes my father from New York before they married, "but I'm anti-suffrage and no arguments I've heard have converted me."

Across the years I am appalled. But there it is in the letter stuffed into the little trunk along with a dance program, souvenirs of the evening when she waltzed the "Golden Sunset" Waltz with Mr. Purdy of DKE at the 1907 Junior Promenade at Hamilton College and the 1903 dance card in which my father is penciled in only for the third two-step and someone has scribbled in the margin, "Would you be true, eyes of blue?"

Old love letters, scarcely recognizable as such, from very proper Cornell and Hamilton boys. Bills for her trousseau—five hats, as per agreement, from a West 47th Street store, $50; and the estimate for the flowers for her wedding—"rather expensive at Christmas, you know," wrote the florist at the bottom of a $100 estimate. And innumerable scrawled notes from me, hoping they would reach my parents before their sailing from various ports of embarkation.

Hats, two-steps, an amused tolerance of the fellow members of her sex fighting for the vote. Not the stuff of which heroines are made. Just a pretty young woman with a quick tongue and no desire to reshape the world. It doesn't do anymore, things are sterner, more is expected of us. There is a certain innocence, like the smell of lavender, rising from these letters.

Ah, but that was earlier, before Dr. Brown and the Santanoni and the cure chair and the Saranac winters that lasted from October through May. The medical diaries were written by a different woman.

Among the old postcards from Palm Beach, the souvenir booklets from Nassau and Haiti, I found a small reflection of another life. Possibly it fell out of the medical diaries, the back pages of which she used for everything from instructions for knitting a sweater to lists of stocks and bonds and recipes for Christmas punch.

Scrawled on the back of a visiting card, she set down the measure of her days:

> write ½ hour
> read ½ hour
> draw ½ hour
> nap 2 hours
> ride 1 hour

I know only the most ordinary things about her. Nothing she has left behind prepares me to understand how she learned to bear, as a matter of course, what was so unbearable.

Eventually she recovered from her setback. The X-rays at Trudeau looked better, and her weight had climbed sixteen pounds to 137 "in galoshes." In March, three months after her tenth wedding anniversary and six months after her temperature had taken off like a skyrocket across the page, Dr. Brown said she might try a trip home for a visit.

Such a thing was not unusual. Once the fever was under control, when bed rest was no longer necessary, the consumptives went about living as nearly normal a life as possible, walking a nervous path in the hope that the sleeping bacilli would not be awakened. The progress of consumption was different with each patient, and its treatment varied with the temperament of the doctor. For whatever reason, Dr. Brown had decided that my mother could try her wings.

I don't believe there was any thought that she was cured. It was only a small milestone, a cautious trial step in the direction of normality. I think Dr. Brown simply decided that she knew enough of the dangers of overdoing and of spreading the infection to her family to be given what amounted to a leave of absence. The period of her sentence was as much in doubt as ever.

Many Saranac consumptives in the twenties lived out their lives in a gray area, neither cured nor bedridden. It is true that some got well and a great many died, but probably by far the largest group lingered as semi-invalids for years. A few were cured of their most virulent symptoms, got fed up with the City of the Sick, chucked it and went home regardless of the doctors.

In the third year of her cure my mother was still obedient to her doctor. She was going home only for a visit, the first time she had set foot in her own home in almost three years. She was not to wear herself out at too many parties, not to overdo the household overseeing. She must promise to rest every possible moment and to observe scrupulously the nap hour. And to retire to her room at the first sign of weariness.

She promised them all anything they asked, but she was already making plans. At last she would see the friends who had not made their way to Saranac in the two and a half years. She would hold my christening, which had been delayed so long I threatened to be a lifelong heathen. And walk in the garden looking for the crocuses she had planted so long ago.

And. . . .

Of course, she said impatiently, already planning what she would wear, she would be careful.

16 ❧

In Rome our household was completely turned upside down. Instructions for my mother's care had arrived in advance of her, and in the kitchen there was much wiping of hands on aprons and polishing of spectacles as they huddled over the typewritten directions. My mother's dishes must be washed separately from the rest, in different water and dishpan. Every glass she drank from must be kept separate, marked with a small piece of adhesive tape at the bottom. Each piece of silver must be tied with a piece of string to identify it as hers and hers alone. Even her salt cellar must be distinctive, square while the rest of the family had round ones.

She must, of course, have her own room. She must go down

and up stairs only twice a day, once for dinner and then once for what we called supper. The household must strictly observe the hours from two to four as quiet hours during which the phone must be kept from ringing, the doorbell silent.

Added to the staff would be a trained nurse, for unless something went wrong my mother would be allowed to stay a month. The nurse would have no care of us children, and, instead of eating in the kitchen, she would expect to eat with the family, unless there were guests.

My mother must take a drive into the country every day and must consume her regular daily six glasses of milk and six eggs. Food must be nutritious and as fattening as possible.

And it would be best if we children spent a minimum of time in her room.

I remember very little of the excitement, but I remember the nurse, who dressed in starchy white and wore a little peaked cap in which I assumed she slept. She actually had very little to do except carry the breakfast tray and innumerable glasses of milk up the back stairs, and she was a thorn in my father's flesh just by being. I can never forget the way his face drooped when he looked at her. I cannot see her face in my mind, only the waves her presence created.

No memory comes to me of my mother's actual arrival. One day she was simply there when I came home from school, lying in a pink chaise longue and smiling. I felt pleased and a little strange. It was another of the large changes in my life about which I had been told nothing.

With her coming, the house took on a life it had never had. Overnight it changed, as if lights had been turned on all over, in every room. You could feel the excitement when you walked up the front steps. People came and went, slamming car doors, laughing and calling back that they would come again soon, leaving small gifts in their wake. The scent of flowers was overpowering in my mother's room. Anna vanished from the living room into the kitchen, and the doorbell and the telephone rang constantly.

At first the ladies were always trooping up the stairs, wafting expensive French perfume and waving gaily over the banister. The nurse regulated their coming and going like a field marshal, ousting them if they overstayed their time. After a week or so, they came in small numbers for supper, at which my mother appeared wearing pretty trailing things and carrying a long cigarette holder. After supper there was Mah-Jongg or bridge, while I sat curled in a corner armchair with a book, trying to get used to having a mother I could have reached out to and touched.

Her temperature stayed within bounds, and the Episcopalian minister was summoned to officiate at my christening. It was a grand occasion with me as the centerpiece, all in white with a pink ribbon in my hair and high white shoes. I had to wear high shoes long after other children had given them up, just as I had to take naps until I was in school all day.

The ceremony took place in the formal parlor. It was relatively painless, involving only a few ritual words and several presents, though the presents were not of the kind I would have selected. Among them were a small silver plate with my name on it and a silver mug embossed with roses and the day of my birth. Afterwards I was excused while my godparents joined the minister in toasting my Christian piety with Manhattan cocktails. While the drinks were making the rounds, the minister excused himself to empty the remains of the holy water under the cedar tree near the front door. I waited until he had gone back to my parents and then I got down on my knees to inspect the spot where he had poured it, but there was nothing at all remarkable about it.

Daily, when the wheels of my father's car scrunched on the gravel of the driveway, my mother descended the stairs to take midday dinner with us. Now that she was there in her chair at the end of the table, delicately rearranging her food on her plate, this familiar meal took on a completely different cast.

A meal which we had eaten briskly and sometimes abstractedly now became a ceremony. A three-course repast was presented from soup to pie, featuring, if not a roast, a substantial meat course expertly carved by my father while Kathleen, in a new cap and apron, stood by to pass. No longer did the vegetables grow cold on the serving table as Kathleen joined in conversation with us children. Food whisked in and out of the kitchen, piping hot in ornate silver dishes, and Kathleen herself suddenly developed a straight-backed dignity which precluded catching my eye. Even the dogs seemed to have better manners, lying quiescent on the new Chinese rug, apparently forgetting to beg.

When the last of the tea had been drunk, my mother would rise and begin the climb to her bedroom, stopping to rest on the landing as Dr. Brown had ordered, the nurse following in her wake with the remains of the milk.

Once back in her room, she remained there behind closed doors until, promptly at four, one or another of her friends' long black cars would draw to a stop at the door and bear her away for a prescribed drive. Not a drive to a destination, but a drive for the sake of driving. To the day he died, my father took a daily drive for pleasure after work. He and my mother came of a generation which could remember when the automobile was not a convenience but a leisure toy.

The house in those weeks of her visit seemed to bulge with

people. I was always peering from the safe haven of the busy kitchen through the swinging door at another formal party, the women with bare shoulders and shiny, high-heeled pumps and the men in black ties and stiff shirts, the room hazy with cigarette smoke, buzzing with conversation. My memory of this time is filled with the sound of their laughter drifting up the stairs to my half-open door as I fell asleep after a meal with Anna in the kitchen.

We might almost for a while have been like other families and my mother like anyone else.

In those weeks that my mother was at home, her circle of friends flocked about her, pretending that there was nothing wrong, nothing worse than a slight indisposition from which she had largely recovered. But outside her set, as they called it, things were different. The house was off limits to many of my friends. Their mothers, though they clucked over me as they might over a recently orphaned child, largely forbade their children our house while my mother was in it.

"My heart breaks for you," said the mother of one of my schoolmates, patting my shoulder as I drank milk and ate cookies in her kitchen.

I stared at her, at pains to conceal my astonishment. I thought perhaps she had somehow found out that I had been one of the last to be chosen for the tug of war at recess.

"Where is your friend Sarah?" inquired Anna carefully one day, busy with my hairbrush, preparing to make a large club of hair on which to mount the ribbon. "I haven't seen her lately."

"She can't come here," I told her reflection in the mirror above my head.

Anna nodded as if she had known it all along, stretching the rubber band about her fingers and pursing her lips.

"I suppose they're afraid," she said primly. "Such a sinful pity, when we're so careful."

I didn't understand her. To a child, his own world is the norm and what happens in it is unquestioned. It never occurred to me to resent the partial social ostracism which was inflicted on me by the parents of my friends during my mother's visit home. I had had a taste of it all my life, the closed looks in the faces of the adults who shook their heads and wouldn't explain when their daughters begged for permission to come to our house to see the current puppy. For there were many who thought the house at any time was dangerous. The world was ruled by adults, and they did as they saw fit.

When I was little, the Department of Health in New York State posted a warning sign on the front door of every household where the doctors reported a contagious disease. A pink placard warned of measles, a yellow one of mumps. I am not sure, but I think there was one for chickenpox. I know there was a red one for scarlet fever, which had not yet been completely conquered. If I thought about our household at all, it was to wonder if there was a card for tuberculosis. I decided that since my mother was only visiting, it wasn't necessary.

Perhaps it was the small town, or the maids, or possibly because it was the age in which one sat on the front porch of a summer day and called to people walking by, but even distant acquaintances seemed to know everything about our household. They spoke to me about our family as if they were intimates of it, discussing it in my presence as if a child were as inanimate as a chair, wouldn't notice, didn't matter. "What a shame," they would cluck, "never to have known a mother. Just home for a visit, isn't she?"

I would nod politely, blocking them out with no effort. I suppose if I had been older when my mother fell ill, I would have contrasted a before and an after and sensed tragedy. I didn't. I had a perfectly good life, if you excused my phobia about tardiness. Adults were and always had been incomprehensible. I studied them covertly when I thought they weren't looking and made allowances for them. They lived by a different set of rules. We were getting along all right.

But my parents knew we were not like anyone else. When Mother had been home a few months, they invited me for what they billed as a ride and a picnic. It turned out to be a long drive through the Cherry Valley to Cooperstown, where we inspected a girls' camp on the lake they had heard about. I trailed about in their wake as the director displayed the boathouse, the craft center, the main lodge and a sample pup tent. After an hour or so, while I was dreamily inspecting the afternoon shadows cast by the pines across the lake, they turned to me and explained brightly that they had enrolled me.

They drove away, waving gaily, leaving me without so much as a toothbrush, not yet six and at a distinct disadvantage, for the camp had already been in session a week.

There is no torture worse than finding yourself at five in the midst of a group all wearing identical brown bloomers and orange scarves you have not got. The LaSalle disappeared down the dirt road in a little poof of dust, and I swallowed the lump in my throat as best I could. They put me in a tent with much older girls, who treated me with enormous contempt, especially after a few days when I injudiciously admitted that Mother signed her letters to me "with gobs of love." I should have known it was the kind of thing you kept to yourself, as you kept it to yourself that you were unhappy. To have a mother unlike others was fatal.

It was the beginning of long years of being farmed out, and

the first and last time I was ever homesick. I stayed to the end of the summer, and when I came home, my mother had gone.

That was the way my life was, and I accepted it, as I accepted the fact that my mother was a bird of passage.

17

I don't think of Mother as especially brave, though she
certainly was no complainer. She loved the good things of life
and was naturally restless in confinement, but she kept this
mostly to herself. Only two or three times in her life do I
remember her referring to what she had to endure over a
period of seventeen years—a form of the rack suffered, it
seems to me a half-century later, with understated grace. All
the way through most of her marriage she lived only a pale
copy of a normal life, but, as far as I know, she never gave up
trying to pretend that this wasn't so. I don't know how much
she counted on an eventual cure. I think she simply refused to
acknowledge, even to herself, the extent of her limitations.

There must have been other moments, but only once can I remember her kicking at the traces. We sat, we four, in the flickering glow of the candles at the table while Kathleen moved among us passing the vegetables. I was drinking my milk and idly contemplating the shadows cast by the candles on the wall across from me when I noticed that Mother's salt cellar was exactly like everyone else's. Not square as usual, but the identical round cut-glass dish that sat at each place.

"Look," I said with the pleased pride of a child who has noticed what the adults have missed, "Mother has the wrong salt cellar."

Kathleen, whose gestures and reactions were always as overdone as those of a minor character in a bad play, halted in her tracks, sucking in her breath with a hand over her mouth.

"I'll change it," she said hastily, abandoning the vegetable she was passing and reaching for the little dish.

But my mother fixed her with a stern eye.

"Leave it," she said, in a tone as cold as the ice in the birdbath outside the window.

And very deliberately she reached for the salt spoon and salted her meat from the wrong dish.

"Bess," said my father gently from the other end of the table. "Bessie, you mustn't."

It was a long time before she met his eye over her plate, and, watching, I had my first glimpse of her tears.

After the first few years I think Mother knew that even if things turned out in the best possible way, the special dishes, the nap, the thermometer and the burden of eating food she didn't want would always be a part of her life. The knack of patience, the adjustment to a time frame as distorted as a reflection in rippling water were arts which she learned because she had to and which eventually became imprinted on her. She accepted a convalescent's life as she had accepted the reality of the disease. She adapted her quicksilver, impulsive ways to the ones imposed on her, as an immigrant adapts to the customs of a new country.

I remember her lying in the big bed in her room early one Christmas morning, the coverlet piled high with gifts. We children had had our own Christmas downstairs early, almost before it was light, and had brought her presents to her, piling them in a heap on the bed.

She was toying with her coffee cup and eyeing the mismash of beautifully wrapped offerings, asking about this and that, smiling and admiring what we brought to show her.

"Open yours," I begged her. "Open the one I gave you," I entreated her, dancing with excitement on the perimeter of the safety line.

She gave me a dazzling smile I can still see, half apologetic and half conspiratorial.

"In a minute," she said over the rim of the coffee cup. "The thinking about it is better than the doing."

Back in Saranac the little leaning tents in the temperature chart seemed better behaved, the four o'clock staying almost at normal. But every so often the pattern traced in sepia ink in the diaries breaks and the fever sets in again, starting at normal and climbing all day. "Sick," she writes in the margin one morning in June. But in a few days the pattern is normal again.

We took the house on Park Avenue for another summer, my mother still remaining in her apartment at the Santanoni. Everything was the way it was before, except that now she could walk a bit farther, do a little more. She had graduated to being treated by Dr. Brown's assistant, Dr. Hayes, and she was allowed to walk to his office in the village, down the long hill and over a block or two.

Once more we were a family of sorts. We had moved, we children, nurses, dogs, my stuffed animals, cartons of books, the whole paraphernalia of our lives, for another summer into the brown-shingled row. From our base in the house we went often to the resorts around us, picnicking, rowing out, all four of us, across the shallows at the edge of Lake Clear, my brother and my father each pulling on an oar. Again we were an island among strangers, a family with roots elsewhere. I can't remember meeting another child in Saranac.

Toward the end of the summer Dr. Hayes said Mother could go with us to Montreal and stay a night or two. It was the first trip away from Saranac except for the visit home, and she was as excited as if it were a safari to Egypt. "Two hundred and seventy miles in the Buick," says the note in the margin of her diary, "new restaurants, new shops, new faces, a new *bed.*" We stayed at the Ritz, sipping tea in the little garden under the British flag which made us feel so far away, climbing part way up Mount Royal in the horse-drawn cabouches while my father called on lumber customers, making small expeditions to stores to buy sweaters. Somehow we had left more than Saranac behind as we peered from the windows of the Buick, giggling at customs officers searching with mirrors under the mudguards for contraband liquor.

"It seems so *foreign,*" said Mother, leaning happily on her elbows at the little table in the Ritz garden, her eyes following the two or three couples enjoying themselves on the terrace dance floor to the strains of the tea-dance orchestra.

"It *is* foreign, Bess," said my father, stirring his tea matter-of-factly.

She threw him an impatient look.

"Why don't you dance with Betty?" she said, still watching the couples drifting about the floor to the staid Ritz music.

I shook my head, but she was smiling at me, humming the words of the tune.

"Don't you want to dance?" she asked, shaking her head in disbelief, but I ducked my own, suddenly shy.

She saw that I meant to sit where I was, and she transferred her gaze to my father, who was meditatively stirring his tea.

"Your daughter doesn't want to dance, but I do," she said suddenly, and then she was on her feet holding out her arms to him.

It was forbidden. We all knew it. She was an invalid to whom even a short walk was an event. But there she was, her little sea-green dress clinging to her thin frame so that it showed the bones of her hips, holding out her arms to him and smiling invitingly.

He didn't say anything at all, to his eternal credit. He simply rose and led her gently onto the dance floor, and they melted into the tiny group of dancers. It was a slow fox-trot and he held her very close, her cheek against his.

After only a minute or so the music broke and he led her back to the table flushed and laughing. When they were once again back in their chairs, he covered her hand with his own, one of the few public gestures of affection I ever saw him make.

"It seems like more than two hundred and seventy miles from Saranac," she said, her eyes on the English flag whipping about in the wind, captive on its standard.

But it wasn't. The limits had only stretched a bit. She was still tethered by a long leash to two or three blocks of a tiny Adirondack village. Her life was still governed by the pulse at her wrist, the heat of her blood. Sick today, better later in the week, movies, a drive, more X-rays.

Improved. But never well.

She was far better off than many lying in the wards of Ray Brook, but this was thin comfort. Time was slipping by, as she stood on the sidelines, the edge between sick and well blurred, but a captive still. With most diseases you fall sick, you get well, it is over. The disease has a recognized course which can be anticipated, counted on, and that is all. In pneumonia, before the drugs, there used to be a dramatic crisis, and if you were lucky, you rose from the bed thankfully with everything behind you, escaped. I remember lying on my stomach on the landing at home while the doctor attended my father in a pneumonia crisis, a common thing before penicillin. You could feel the tension seeping out from under the door of the room where the doctor bent over him. People stepped over me without noticing me, bearing trays and looking distraught. Nobody said so, but I knew he might die. For a day or two the household held its breath, and then suddenly it was over and he was on the road to recovery.

But tuberculosis, the most feared of the diseases, had no such sharp outlines, no prognosis, no course to run. In the sanitariums spread about the village from Hemorrhage Hill to the Riverside Inn lay hundreds of patients confined to bed who had no idea at all when, or even if, they would rejoin the world. To these patients, the doctor's word was like that of Moses handing down the Ten Commandments. There were no patterns, no guidelines; everything depended on what the medical men said. To the consumptive, the doctor was jailer, priest, confidant, miracle worker, friend and God, all rolled into one magnificent, omniscient being.

They are all gone now, every one of the doctors who were part of the early cure days in Saranac, stumbling along in a field in which so little was known. They were pioneers hampered by the ignorance of the times, yet there is nothing to match them today. In the tiny kingdom of Saranac founded by Edward Trudeau, they were the nobility, and *noblesse oblige*. Dr. Edward Trudeau's telephone number was 1, and it was symbolic. His grandson, Dr. Francis Trudeau, Jr., says that to be a Trudeau when he was small was to be one step above the village priest. Even beyond the limits of Saranac the Trudeau name was so respected that the family got ten percent off when they bought clothing in Montreal and young Frank got a reduction at St. Paul's School when he attended. Later, when he returned to practice medicine in his grandfather's house, fear of TB had passed into history and he had to surmount town-and-gown animosity. But in the twenties, to be a doctor in Saranac was to be a Brahmin, and to be called Trudeau was to have been born to the purple.

They were mortal and they made mistakes, but in many ways they deserved the homage they received. They were dedicated in a way that is hard to imagine in these days when the house call is only a memory and if you need to see your doctor you'd better plan a week ahead. They were brilliant men, combining the research and practice which are so rigidly separated today, and they cared deeply about curing tuberculosis. They were the reason the consumptives clung to hope.

My mother, in her indeterminate sentence, was relying on the most famous doctor outside the Trudeaus themselves, a man who, if the Trudeaus were royalty, might have been their prime minister. Of all the doctors, Dr. Brown was perhaps the most sympathetic—a nervous man with a baffling skin ailment who, even when he and his wife had guests for dinner, kept the telephone by his chair at the table.

"We thought that a bit much," says Mrs. Kinghorn now, but to the patients on the other end it was a lifeline. Lawrason Brown had contracted TB when he was in his third year at Johns Hopkins, and he understood.

But then so did others. Dr. Kinghorn suffered a hemorrhage on duty at Montreal General Hospital and arrived in Saranac, like so many others, on a stretcher. All of them, with only one or two exceptions, knew first hand how it felt. Dr. Edward R. Baldwin, who eventually took over the reins from Dr. Edward Trudeau, rang Dr. Trudeau's doorbell one frosty morning and announced that he had TB and asked to be admitted to Trudeau Institute. He had identified his own disease with his microscope. It is a measure of how many desperate consumptives flocked to Saranac that Baldwin had to wait six weeks to be admitted.

Dr. J. Woods Price (a Virginian who became young Frank Trudeau's godfather), Dr. Charles C. Trembley (who at the turn of the century became resident physician at Trudeau), dapper Dr. Edgar Mayer, Dr. Sidney F. Blanchet, Dr. Edward Packard—all of them had personally felt consumption's ravages. Among the famous doctors, only John Hayes, assistant to Dr. Brown, escaped.

They conferred biweekly in the John Black Memorial across from the Kinghorn house on Church Street, and they took seriously the fact that consumptives from all over the world had come to them for the cure. Even on Sunday they cranked up their Franklins if they were needed, and they suffered with grace the intrusions of relatives of their patients on their private weekend life. The Sunday dinner, the usual cold spread in the evening, were interrupted hours for them almost every week.

If they kept largely to themselves socially at dinner dances at the Pines, at the card tables, on the golf course, it was because they were closer than brothers. It was their town, their snowy kingdom for which they had left metropolitan centers. They never locked their doors, their cars were familiar to everyone they passed, they were bowed to and pointed out when they attended services at the Church of St. Luke the Beloved Physician. *"My* doctor," says each recovered patient living on in Saranac today, "was a wonderful man—the best." And each may be speaking of a different great man.

Still it was no wonder they felt as they did, remember a father figure with skilled hands. To these early doctors, the tubercular bacillus was the most fascinating creature in the world, and they begrudged no time spent trying to conquer it. They had left rich practices to live in an isolated country town where the streets were cleared by horse-drawn plows, and not one of them would have considered doing anything else. Most stayed on to die there. For them it was the center of the world. They were fighting in the first lines the greatest killer in the United States.

They lived well and loved their adopted village.

"It was so gay," says Mrs. Kinghorn. "It was like wine just to breathe the air."

Mrs. Kinghorn's house on Church Street had nine bedrooms and two maids' rooms. Dr. Trudeau's, as befitted the founder, was a charming, inviting New England type with an office tastefully furnished with mementoes of his sportsman outings. Dr. Price's house on Main Street, just around the corner from Church, had an entrance flanked by four white pillars which reminded him of his native Virginian style of architecture. Elegant to his fingertips, Dr. Price carried a gold-headed cane and a gold thermometer case.

Dr. Trembley was the acknowledged prince of the yarn spinners, but it was Dr. Mayer who had the richest patients, the most adulation. The ladies loved Dr. Mayer, who had various movie-star patients out at the Will Rogers sanitarium and at whose house Grace Moore was often a guest. There are those who say they shut up the sanitarium when he stopped practicing, so much did it depend on him.

Dr. Edward Welles lived up the hill on Church Street, just before Catherine Street, the dividing line between the chic and the not so chic. It was he who invented the operation called thoracoplasty, and his patients were recognizable on the streets by the way they listed slightly from the surgery. He later invented a small sandbag to balance them better.

These were the great men.

"Our little dinners were so jolly and bright," sighs Mrs. Kinghorn. "It's so dead now. It was so different after the cities, the way we didn't lock our doors. But then, of course, lots of people wouldn't have cared to come near us."

Lots of people wouldn't. But the better-known doctors looked on the risk as part of the game. They scrubbed up carefully before going home after the day with the patients, and they forbade their children to attend Saranac movies. But on the whole they were sanguine about the risks. They were as careful as possible, and after that, what could anyone do? Frank Trudeau says he was never allowed to come to his father's office, and he still remembers Dr. Trudeau, senior, driving home with only his little fingers guiding the steering wheel because he had not yet had an adequate wash-up.

But the old gentleman never had a chest X-ray till he suffered a heart attack at sixty-five.

In an odd sort of way, it may have been medicine's finest hour. Medicine was not a living for these men, it was their life. When they weren't actually tending the sick, or bending over the microscope slides, they were fund-raising. Trudeau Institute was built from philanthropic funds.

Their patients came straight to their doorsteps from the

train depot, clutching scraps of paper with the name of the illustrious man scribbled in pencil.

The legend of Saranac's fame is laced with unbelievable true stories. On a train rolling west sometime during the twenties a man seated in the diner began to cough. Walking past him in the aisle, a woman hearing him came to a dead stop in her tracks.

"You have consumption, don't you?" she said, turning to look at him.

He admitted that he did and was en route to Arizona for his health.

She looked at him incredulously.

"Don't you know," she said, placing a kindly hand upon his shoulder, "that Saranac is the only place in the country to get well? Get off this train at the next station, take a train back where you came from and go to Saranac. When you get there, take a taxi to Dr. Lawrason Brown's house. He'll know what to do."

That's the way they came to Saranac Lake in the early days, as this man eventually did. Someone had told them the great doctors would help them. Nothing else, including money, really mattered.

The doctors walked the streets of Saranac a little less than gods, but sometimes they were strangely innocent. Eddie Diamond was a patient of Dr. Francis Trudeau, and right up to the end the good doctor never knew who he was.

After each visit Eddie would reach under his mattress for a fat roll of bills to peel off enough to pay. Sometimes he gave Trudeau enough to pay the sanitarium on the way out, and the doctor always obliged.

When Trudeau eventually had to sign Eddie's death certificate, he was puzzled by the presence of two burly men who obviously packed guns, flanking the bedside respectfully.

He inquired who they were.

"Read the morning papers," said the taller of the two through barely moving lips. And indeed it was not until the morning paper hit the Trudeau stoop that the doctor discovered he had been attending a notorious underworld character.

Possibly it was not innocence which kept Dr. Trudeau unaware of the underworld, but preoccupation. For these doctors there were no office hours, their work expanded through their waking hours. When they were not actually attending their patients, they were very often advising and comforting them.

"I am going home soon for good," my mother told Dr. Brown one frigid winter day, avoiding his eye. "Well or not."

Whatever he told her kept her there another year. But she was pulling at the tether. Rebellion was a small but growing seed. The trip home had left her dissatisfied, tired of waiting.

Among her things I found a faded postcard of an old barn standing square against the rural hills which form a backdrop to the five combines of the old barge canal near Rome.

"If earth has a region of bliss," she has written on the sky above the barn, "it is this, it is this."

She really meant to go home before long.

18 ❧

She was up nearly to 140 pounds, more than twenty pounds heavier than she was the day my father first brought her to Saranac.

"I'm fat," she said in disgust over her shoulder to my father, turning this way and that in front of the mirror to see the whole truth.

"It's like insurance, Bess," my father told her gently, thinking she hadn't looked better since he brought her to Saranac.

Her lower lip was curled in scorn at her own reflection.

"It's the beer," she said finally, tugging at her belt. "They're always suggesting another glass."

She flung herself suddenly into the chair by the bedside, staring over his shoulder at the mountain beyond him.

"I won't stay much longer, you know," she said. "I've had my fill of the snow and the mountains."

They were treating her with a sun lamp now, and she looked round and healthy, the way she had looked when he first met her. Well, plumper, of course. But by Saranac standards it was a small gain.

"You look lovely, Bess," said my father, and he meant it.

Perhaps it was the hair that troubled her. It was funny about the hair. It had gone white almost overnight, the way they say it does in books when you have a narrow escape or bad news. The change had been so quick, there was so little in-between gray—one day the gold hair and then the white. My father's head had scarcely a gray hair, and my mother was eight years younger.

"You're not paying any attention to me," she complained.

She was right. He had been wondering where to add the sleeping porch to their home in Rome. She would be coming home soon. There would be no keeping her much longer.

She was at the mirror now, running a comb through the offending white locks.

"I'd like to go to dinner somewhere very nice," she said, and he heard the catch in her voice.

He put his arms around her, feeling the bones of her ribs against his chest.

"Get your coat," he said into her ear. "I'm taking you to a new place they told me about at the hotel."

At least he could do that for her.

There were plenty of new places. This was 1927, the apex of Saranac's fame, and whatever it had been seven years ago when she arrived was now doubled in spades. Saranac was riding high, bulging with more and more new arrivals who had heard the word of the cure center and the brilliant doctors.

They were pouring into Saranac, and more rooms were needed. William Scopes, sensing that the moment was right, had opened his new Hotel Saranac just behind Dr. Trudeau's house on Main Street; it was the first fireproof edifice in the Adirondacks and some said the finest north of New York City. No expense had been spared. The lobby was a replica of the foyer in the Davanzati Palace in Florence. Every one of its hundred rooms had a bath. The exposed beams in the lobby were painted in the Italian manner, and the massive stone fireplace was carved with figures which appeared in the Davanzati coat of arms.

The lobby rode a story above the street to discourage casual walk-ins and, some whispered, tubercular patients. Its advertisements specified "no consumptives," but its hundred rooms were constantly full of their relatives and some who coughed in the night. Evenings the guests dined in the paneled dining room under elegant chandeliers. Saranac in the twenties had come a long way from a north-country trading post.

Scopes spent $750,000 on the hotel. A couple of years later, when the market crashed, he was overextended and nearly went broke.

But this was 1927, the market was behaving like a Roman candle, the sky was the limit, gin was easy to come by and there was no tomorrow, especially in Saranac. My mother had her hair marcelled and finger-waved, and on her birthday my father brought her a little braided gold-mesh bracelet studded with diamonds. The New York Central was a vital link for the East and rode at least partially on my father's railroad ties. Even with the expenses of the Santanoni, he could afford a new LaSalle. He drove it frequently, when the weather was good, up the back road from Rome to Montreal and Quebec, where his purchasing sources were, stopping in Saranac to see Mother, take her out on the town, for a drive, to a curling match.

It was an even harder-drinking village than it had been seven years ago. There was plenty of expensive liquor in the speaks and plenty in the restaurants. Through the Saranac Hotel arcade you could see St. Bernard's Catholic Church, designed by the stonemason Pete Tanzini. At the Santanoni, Tanzini's name was well known, but not from any church-going. On the side, Tanzini was the king of the Saranac bootleggers, the hard stuff where the money was. In a garage at the edge of town crouched Pete's eight souped-up Packards and Cadillacs, ready to make the nightly run across the border. His cars were fleet and his operations skilled, and stonemasonry became a sideline. But two years later he was to answer the doorbell in his bedroom slippers, open the door to a stranger and disappear forever. A few days after his disappearance his wife received a telephone call—the operator documents the time—hung up and went upstairs and shot herself. But in 1927, none of this had yet occurred, and half the guests at the Riverside Inn and the Pines owed a debt of gratitude to Pete Tanzini.

It was Saranac's zenith. A hundred private sanitariums were keeping full beds, as was St. Mary's of the Lake, a sanitarium run by the Sisters of Mercy on Ampersand Avenue. Out on the road to Placid, the National Variety Artists Association Lodge had moved from a Park Avenue house to another imposing Scopes edifice dedicated to the care of consumptive stage and screen stars as well as lesser members of the industry. The public rooms were as lavish as Hollywood sets, the walls hung with portraits of cinema greats. Even the smallest rooms looked out on a magnificent panorama of mountains. Out at Stoney Wald, the New York Telephone Company maintained a less elegant sanitarium for the exclusive use of female consumptives.

Money was easy, and plenty of it came into Saranac. The town was swinging wide and high, with nightclub acts from Montreal playing every weekend in the Mount Baker Club and the streets full of Pierce Arrows, Cadillacs and Duesenbergs. Hair and skirts were short, like the life expectancy of some of the residents, who, while they could, meant to make each day count. The speaks were jammed, and the Pontiac played to standing room only. Jack Dempsey, King of the Ring, was training at the St. Regis. On the Fourth of July, William Morris brought a carload of Broadway names from New York, with starlets in fake sleighs carrying marabou muffs, to perform for everybody ambulatory.

Mrs. Frank Trudeau, playing cards with friends, was not above mentioning Trudeau's need for funds. Birthday and Christmas cards arrived at the Trudeau home stuffed with gift checks for the sanitarium, at least one of them bearing a windfall donation in four figures. Everybody said it was the most lavish since Dr. Edward Trudeau made a house call to Murray Bay, sent a bill for $50 and received a check for $5,000. "Your bill was outrageous," said the accompanying note.

Everything was as profligate and sybaritic, as frenetic and oddly innocent as the twenties themselves. My mother, watching from the cure chair on her sleeping porch, was determined to leave it all behind.

Restless as she was, it was harder than it had ever been

before to lie in her chair docilely working the crossword puzzle in the *Herald Tribune* while the little radio beside her beat out the songs everybody else was dancing to. She knew all the words to every one of them. She read, knitted, stared at the mountains from her cure chair, wrote letter after letter. Sometimes she put the books away and got out her paintbox to do some quiet watercolor drawings that my father brought home to us—fashionable ladies leaning over balustrades, looking not unlike herself.

The days were longer than they had ever been.

When she got home, she decided, she would have the piano tuned.

At home we had long ago grown used to a life without her.

"How is your mother?" friends of the family would inquire when they met me walking with the dogs or trudging home from school.

"Fine," I would assure them.

How would I know? I, least of all. My father scarcely spoke of her condition. We children were an antidote to her illness, a buffer from loneliness. I tagged after him when he went to have his shoes shined, sat beside him on the high bench while the shoeshine boy expertly performed his miracles with a snapping cloth and an abstracted whistle. I remember trailing after him on countless visits to his maiden sister who lived in his boyhood home, or waiting for him while he played golf so we could take a drive together. He liked knowing I was there, having me with him, but he wanted to talk about anything but Mother.

What a curious pair we must have made, we constant companions—me with my haircut from his barber and my boy's suit stolen from my brother, he the glass of fashion, handsome, abstracted. We never did anything suitable for children. He just kept me by him in his life.

There were plenty of women, widows and divorcees, who would have been delighted to help him pass the time, but it was I who shared his after-work hours. We had a regular beat, he and I: the newsstand, the market, the country club. He had his own thoughts, and I was accustomed to that. It was a quiet, undemanding companionship that I think helped him.

Years later I remember standing at the funeral of my husband, staring chin up and dry-eyed at the proceedings when an acquaintance passed behind me.

"It's all right to cry, you know," she whispered in my ear.

Nobody in our family thought so. Whatever we knew of each other, we knew through a kind of osmosis. Emotions, worries, complaints were bad form. Personal reticence was much the fashion in my parents' circle.

"Will your mother be coming home soon?" the librarian asked me as I deposited my armful of books on her desk.

"Oh, yes," I told her. "Quite soon."

Actually, her return was still some time away. It was always understood to be soon, but never scheduled. She always seemed to be in the wings, part of the family but missing. She was someone I wrote to, was related to, but with whom my acquaintance was slight. In her presence all my early childhood, I was polite and slightly constrained.

Sorting through memories of my moments alone with her, I am appalled at the yawning void across which we spoke.

"How is school?" she would begin tentatively, like a courtesy auntie come to call, anxious to ingratiate.

"Fine."

I am likewise anxious to be friendly, but not sure how. I affect to be studying the collection of glass animals on her bureau.

"I made a list of the Hit Parade songs last night from the radio," she says. "It's there on the chair."

We share an interest in dance tunes. I thank her and put it in my pocket and make my way to the door.

"Stand up straight, darling," she calls, and I am gone.

It never crossed my mind that she needed me.

Years later, when the Santanoni was only an elegant burnt-out shell, I asked if I could go upstairs to look around. The owner led me up the blackened stairwell, cautioning me to mind the loose boards, to a suite of rooms which I thought I remembered.

But I might never have stood there, a small girl with high white shoes, trying to make the lady on the bed into my mother. It was all wrong, nothing remained in that desolate room that smelled of smoke. I was there more than once, perhaps several times, I see it in my mind's file, but I could not fit us into what he showed me. It was all too long ago; only my father came here regularly. It was impossible to think of this room full of flowers, of white-capped nurses and elegant women in marabou-trimmed negligees, crossing silken-clad legs and sipping sherry.

"Do you remember it?" asked the owner, standing against a singed partition, testing its weight.

"No," I told him, and we went down the blackened staircase together in silence.

She was only 150 miles from us in Saranac, but she might have been a thousand. The backroads to Saranac over Elmer

Hill, Blue Mountain and Otter Lake were frightening in the winter, and my father almost always went to Utica to take the train through endless forest land to Lake Clear Junction, where he changed for the Saranac-Placid spur. We children stayed at home in the winter. I don't remember how she looked in the Santanoni.

But then I don't remember how she looked in her bed at home, speaking to me across the length of the big room.

Childhood is always abstracted, obsessed with its own problems, unaware that adults could possibly have their own. You have only to run through the pages of old photo albums to see how much we miss as children. Can this young woman, forever in this picture so much younger than I, be my mother? Is this thin, handsome man leaning against a pillar and scowling into the sun the man I trudged after all my childhood?

We never really look at our parents until we are grown and they are old. We pack away mental slides of moments involving them, a sort of frozen glimpse of how it was then. Children do not see, they feel, are caught instantly when the vibrations of the room alter, but they miss appearances. Until we develop our own protective shell, essential for dealing with the world, we are tuned like a wild channel to unspoken words, suppressed fear, incipient drama. The cast of characters are stock figures labeled Mother, Father, Cook.

But every detail of how the front parlor looked and felt at the exact moment we discovered that my brother had caught consumption is engraved on my mind.

19

We are sitting, my brother and I, in the long formal parlor of our house waiting for supper. He is in the big leather chair my father brought from his old home, a chair worn, scuffed, accustomed to my father's contours and totally out of place amid the Louis XVI gilded tables and cabinets, the Empire sofas my mother had inherited to furnish the room. In the corner of the blue velvet settee a supply nurse sits sewing. She is there, I remember, because Anna is visiting her sister-in-law for a few days and my father needs someone besides the maids to watch over the household.

I am deep in Albert Payson Terhune, choking back the tears at some terrible cruelty to one of the collies. We all—

including Joe, the fat black cocker idly scratching an ear on the hearth rug—await the call to supper.

My father has just come in, bringing with him the sharp late-fall cold outside. He is poking the fire and inquiring about our day when, thwack, the *Rome Daily Sentinel* hits the front stoop with the evening delivery and my brother is on his feet to fetch it.

Idly we listen to his progress through the vestibule door, through the storm porch to the steps and back again, preceded by an icy gust of cold air.

"Anything in the paper?" asks my father, and my brother stands, tilting the headlines to the light from the fringed lamp on the table.

I have returned to Bruce's peregrinations in search of home and master when something about the stillness of the room makes me look up. The nurse is standing beside my brother's chair, the flat of one hand to his forehead, her sewing suspended in the other. My brother—a serious, small boy wearing knickers and glasses—is looking up at her uneasily, the paper drooping unnoticed to his lap.

It is all there distilled forever, the moment when we knew he, too, had caught tuberculosis. The film runs off the reel at this precise moment and I lose the thread, but this picture is etched in my mind. It couldn't have been anything but a suspicion—something, I think, to do with the way his small errand had winded him—but the air crackled with foreboding. Did they take his temperature, call the doctor, eat supper trying to pretend nothing was wrong? I only see him looking up at the nurse, the newspaper ignored, that uneasy look on his face.

He was fourteen and I ten, and things were never quite the same again for any of us. Certainly not for him, who to this day walls the ensuing months off, seals them like a room shut off to conserve heat in a cold house. Certainly not for my father who now had two invalids to provide for—or for my mother, twisting and turning at night, wrestling with the burden of guilt, no matter how they tried to reassure her.

And also not for me, for when our lives had all been rearranged, I never saw that house again except as a visitor. What had happened to my brother could easily happen to me. Increasingly I became a denizen of dormitory halls, pup tents, and schoolmates' guest bedrooms.

"I would like to help you, but you have inquired into an area that is closed," says my brother when I ask him to tell me how it was. It is rather as if he had committed some terrible crime, paid his debt to society and started a new life.

He went to Saranac almost immediately. Pleurisy, they said, a small spot on the lung. Maybe they only called it pleurisy as people today still often avoid putting a name to cancer with all its terrible implications. "Oh, they kept it very quiet," says a friend who knew us then. There may even have been a few who were left with the impression he was away at school.

It is difficult now to remember how enormously feared a diagnosis of TB was in the twenties. For decades now cancer has been the specter in the wings, the disease for which we employ euphemisms and the possibility of which haunts anyone with any imagination. Cancer is another word for terminal—a killer that claims fewer victims than heart attacks, but is far more terrifying. It is the disease which denies hope, one against which the doctors usually fight only a delaying battle.

In the twenties all these horrors came with tuberculosis. My brother's illness was double disaster, and our family and those nearest to us closed ranks—if not actually to conceal, them to downplay.

I'm not sure, but I think my father rented a house for my mother and brother to live in in Saranac. I am not sure of much of anything that happened shortly after that, for we became almost like two separate families, my father and I the well ones, my mother and brother living through an extended nightmare, wrapped in their blanket cocoons in cure chairs in the bitter Saranac winter.

My sister-in-law tells me that each time she and my brother drove through Saranac in later years he would make a detour past that house, slowing down, leaning out to stare silently at a piece of his life about which he will not speak. In the photo album there are pictures of him wearing a hat with earflaps, mittens and a scarf, looking round and healthy and quiescent in his cure chair, reading with his back to the house. I think he studied on his own, trying to make up the year he missed at school.

Nothing brought the impact of TB home to me like the sight of my brother lying there wrapped like a mummy in a blanket, immobilized, turning the pages with mittened hands. No longer did they have to tell me to wash my hands. For here before my eyes was proof that what had seemed a meaningless ritual carried built-in punishment for those who failed to perform it. Fear of TB became an obsession with me.

At the school I was attending at the time, they took the usual health histories. "Anyone in the family suffer from a serious communicable disease?" asked the busy nurse, pencil poised. I was without guile. I told them everything, and the resulting excitement stunned me. It was only defused by a promise from my father to seek a clean bill of health for me from a prominent specialist. I was hauled off to Saranac, quivering with anxiety, for an X-ray and a going-over by Dr. Brown.

I was, quite simply, terrified. I was convinced, I knew in my bones that I too had the disease. But as long as it was not documented, I could still deny it. They had to physically haul me along the sidewalk to the X-ray office. There was no question in my mind that what had happened to my brother and mother would happen to me. I saw myself in the third cure chair, my lungs a mass of cavities. My father's face beside me didn't reassure me.

But I was returned to school certified harmless, and I vowed to stay that way.

Not surprisingly, my father watched my health anxiously. Every cold was looked upon with grave foreboding, for my mother's illness had come on after a cold. My slightest cough drew alarmed looks: the cough was the visible sign of TB. I had a lot of colds, and every one was a matter of uneasy discussion. Was I drinking my milk? Did I feel that I was improving, or did I think I had a fever? I learned to cough when my father was not present. His worry crippled me.

Once we were driving north together to see Mother and my brother at a time when I was suffering one of my perpetual colds. Closeted alone with my father in a car for five hours, I did not see how I could avoid a bad time. I invented a game to conceal my rather terrifying cough.

"Am I laughing or crying?" I would ask my father innocently, burrowing my face between my hands into the car upholstery and letting loose with a cough that would have panicked him.

He played the game patiently without ever suspecting, and I felt I had made an escape.

But the fear was building in me, brick by brick, bolstered

by the constant worry, by the realization of what it meant to contract TB. I refused to read anything about the disease, I left the room if they spoke of it, did my schoolwork with the specter of the disease always peering over my shoulder. I imagined the taste of blood in my mouth, anxiously gauged my hunger to check loss of appetite, woke in the night in a cold sweat I knew was the fever breaking, so common a symptom of TB.

I had phthisiphobia—the dread of tuberculosis. The whole country in the twenties had phthisiphobia, but it completely possessed me. I was a grown woman and my mother had been dead more than a decade before the very word tuberculosis ceased to paralyze me and I broke the fear's hold on me.

✿ 20

Now it was not just my mother but my brother whom we went to visit, my father and I. The division grew even more pronounced between the sick and the well in our family. They were two who spoke a language we did not, rather as if they knew something we never could. My father and I bumbled about them like children who meant well but were rather too bumptious, regaling them with small stories of life elsewhere. They were members of a secret society, gazing without rancor but with little interest at outsiders who could never be anything else.

They were patient with us, but we were not like them, not so interesting or so complicated. In my brother's eyes, my permanent handicap of youth was now compounded by my rude good health. My father, laboring under the necessity for making a living, had not so much time as they for the literary world. He preferred the golf course and could not discuss Thornton Wilder or e. e. cummings. E. M. Cloran, the Nietzsche follower, begins his essay on sickness with the sentence, "Whatever his merits, a man in good health is always disappointing." I did not understand that then, but it is clear to me now.

My recollection of this period is spotty, for I was left at home as much as possible when Father visited them, kept as much as possible from double exposure to their germs. I lived now in a world populated by Anna, the cook (whose name escapes me) and Kathleen. I sat with them as they drank their endless cups of tea at the gate-leg table in the kitchen, absorbing their views on life, sharing their dreams of amassing enough money to buy a car and retire to Jacksonville, Florida, and play Bingo every night. When my father was in residence, I moved to the seat on his right in the dining room, dining by candlelight and waited on by my companions of the week before. We labored through a three-course meal complete with fingerbowls with floating blossoms, while he told me stories of his boyhood when he and his friends—RoyEdwardsArthurCarpenterFredKessingerTeddyComstock—he always said them in one long breath—fished in muddy creeks, knelt to find Indian arrowheads, waked each other early by twitching a string connected to a big toe and hung out the window.

We did not talk about TB.

I was accustomed to my mother's absence, but it was unsettling to see my brother's empty place at the table. My father redoubled his efforts to keep me well, ordering a pitcher of milk at the ready beside my place at every meal, urging another scarf, an early bedtime. Every other week he filled the house with my mother's friends, who put their arms around me and inquired what I needed, consulted with Kathleen over the linen and silver and complimented the cook on the food until she went pink with pleasure. Alternate weeks I lived with the servants while he pursued his business in New York City.

Their talk of tuberculosis riveted me to my chair. They were a bottomless mine of misinformation, though I wasn't so sure at the time.

The cook thought you couldn't get it if you were fat, and she patted her ample stomach with satisfaction. "It's like a lucky charm," she said, "being fat."

The others weren't so positive. They had heard tell that things were more dangerous in warm weather. And books were especially dangerous. Germs were breathed on them. It was a good thing to wash your hands frequently, but you had to be careful of books.

I didn't really believe any of this, although I didn't say so, but it was the kind of thing I thought about when I woke up at night.

And then suddenly, just as I had grown accustomed to living in a strange divided world, my mother and brother both came home for good. I have no idea how it happened, what decisions were made out of my earshot, though I know my brother was mending fast. I think now that my mother had simply finally had enough. Quite without warning one day, the lease on the Saranac house was canceled and we were told they were both coming home.

I asked my father later how it all came about, and he simply shook his head.

"It broke my heart," he said, "to have your brother put his

arms around my neck and beg to come home. And your mother had been there too long."

Their coming was heralded by frenzied activity. The house was to be made over with a complete new wing for my mother and a sleeping porch for each of them. A nurse and a chauffeur would be hired, and Anna would retire. The house would be converted into a private version of a sanitarium for two.

Carpenters arrived, swarming over the house with their measures, their lathes and their joists. A porch grew on top of the front storm porch, so that the house itself looked unfamiliar when I came up the front steps. Over the driveway a second sleeping porch bulged, opening into a large new bedroom with its own bath and back stairs to the kitchen. An Adirondack cure chair arrived from Saranac; electricians ran wires for a bell to the kitchen, where everybody was in a permanent state of anticipation. The phone rang constantly, and the dogs spent their days attempting to ferret out the new places the workmen had left their sandwiches.

A new second maid was added and set to work polishing the silver kept separate for my mother and sewing tape on the towels which would be hers. While he was about it, my father hauled in several loads of dirt and bricked over the top for a terrace where my mother and brother could sit before and after meals.

"So she's coming home," they said to me, smiling, in Sunday school, in the library, in the candy store where I spent my collection-plate money on licorice whips.

I would nod solemnly. I was a little nervous about the idea. Mother had been gone a long time, and my brother was a stranger.

Again I wasn't there when they arrived and John, the

chauffeur, carried Mother upstairs to her new bedroom while my father ensconced my brother on his porch. She was lying on the chaise longue when I came home from school, and when she saw me she reached out her arms in a convulsive little gesture while I sidled up to her chair, uncomfortably aware of seeming stiff.

"How do you like my new room?" she asked encouragingly, one thin arm encircling my waist, the other rearranging my hair. "It's rather splendid, don't you think? I'm going to have a fire right away in the fireplace."

I could only nod, struck dumb with the importance of the occasion, of having a mother in residence, all the time, forever.

"Are you glad to see me?" she asked, settling back in the chair, and I nodded, unable to look at her.

When she leaned nearer again, adjusting the hair ribbon in my hair, I held my breath.

"Is there anything in the world you want that I can get you?" inquired my father, looking at my brother reclining on his new porch.

"A parrot," he said.

Rome could not produce a parrot, but after a long search one was discovered in Utica and took up residence in the sewing room, whose windows gave on my brother's porch. It was far too cold for the parrot on the porch, but my brother could watch him all day in his cage on the sewing machine, living a querulous, greedy life largely unaware of his observer.

Trays were constantly going up and down the back stairs, the doorbell was always ringing and the house, after months of empty bedrooms, seemed bursting at the seams. Someone was always arriving with groceries, flowers, books. People came and went, but I missed Anna, who had retired to her little brick house near the center of town. I took to going there after school, sitting at her oilcloth-covered dining-room table and helping her mix batches of cookies.

Mornings when I woke I could hear my mother in her bathroom, the window of which angled out from mine, coughing. It was a deep, frightening cough which I could never reconcile with my delicate-looking mother. The cough was one of the sounds I woke to, like the whir of a neighbor's hand mower or the sound of the hammer on a new house workmen were building in the vacant lot down the street. She coughed only in the morning, or I heard it only then, and at first it frightened me. Later I grew accustomed to it. It became a household sound like bathwater running before breakfast or the clinking of dishes in the kitchen when the day was beginning. But all her bright smiles over the breakfast tray when I went in to say hello before going to school could not erase the memory of that cough.

Very soon my brother was on his feet again. How soon I am not sure, because one evening very shortly after the arrival of the invalids, my father slipped his arm around my waist, put down his paper and murmured over my head to my mother as if I weren't present, "She's old enough to go away to school."

Two weeks later I was wedged into the back seat of the car between my parents and once more en route to Cooperstown. Just to look, they said reassuringly, just think how close it is. It astonishes me now how little I felt then, how incurious I sat between them awaiting their decision on where I would spend my life. I trailed after them docilely as we inspected a drafty dining hall, a gym pungent with the smells of gyms everywhere and endless corridors with doors opening off them. After a while my mother went out and sat in the back of the car and I followed her. Nobody seemed to care where I went, and I stood in the weak sunshine by the car window feeling a little forlorn.

"Would you like to stay here?" my mother asked after a while, rolling down the window and peering out at me from under her big hat.

"Without a uniform?" I cried in alarm. I had known a uniformless two weeks at camp. But she only shook her head.

When I saw the bright smile on the face of the portly woman emerging from the school's front door with my father, I knew I would stay without a uniform, without so much as a toothbrush again. They drove off, waving cheerfully, promising to visit in two weeks. So close, they kept saying, leaning from the window.

I scarcely heard them.

"I'd like a roommate, please," I said, peering up at the headmistress.

I thought it would make it easier to borrow a nightgown.

I was eleven years old, but I had already learned the basics of survival away from home.

They telephoned me every two or three days. I can still hear the call for me hallooing down those drafty corridors as I sat studying my Latin in my room. The dogs were all right, Ed would be going to Andover soon, he was better and better, though he had lost a year of school. Was the food good? Was I eating properly? Had the headmistress had her hair done yet? (This from Mother.)

I went home for weekends occasionally, picked up and driven home by John. I sat beside him in my uniform, complete with polo coat and navy-blue beret, peering out at the Cherry Valley slipping by the window as he sang to me in his lovely Welsh lyric tenor. Nelson Eddy was his hero, and he knew all of his songs, along with a huge repertoire of thundering ballads like "The Road to Mandalay." I loved to hear him sing, and we became close friends.

He kept me advised of all the news. My mother was doing well, my brother had left for school. Kathleen had had trouble with her teeth, the collie with mange. It was possible he might win the city bowling tournament.

I heard it all from a comfortable distance. They had managed at last to move my center elsewhere. I was wondering as he spoke if I would make the lower-school hockey team.

❧ 21

"I believe you are most fortunate in getting a fellow like Ted," wrote my mother's brother, Frank, to her on her honeymoon in the Florida Keys. "He is a pretty fine sort and has a wonderful disposition, so look out for your own. We all have our faults and it is pretty near up to the individual whether our path is strewn with roses or thorns. How is that for a sermon?"

I imagine my mother laughing and tossing his letter aside, putting on her big hat in the mirror, ready to walk out in the sun beside my father. But in the unending course of hundreds of meals, I sat between her and my father, longing to defend him while she put that wonderful disposition to the test. She was a great tease, sharp sometimes, I think with private desperation, subject to black moods, pouting, teasing him for his eye for a pretty woman, his predilection for movie magazines. Andover and Yale had failed to make an intellectual out of him, and his bedtime reading was light and brief. "His only books were women's looks and folly all they taught him," my mother would say to nobody in particular, drumming her slim fingers on the table and rearranging the silver.

He never answered her back, gentling her like a high-spirited horse, though he was sometimes annoyed with others. "That horrible mess in regard to your wedding carriage was not really my fault as Ted seems to think," protested my Uncle Frank in a scrawled letter from his law offices. But for his Bess my father never had a sharp word. I think he understood that she carried invisible wounds as much as any veteran of a shooting war.

Dr. Brown said the nervous system in TB was affected by the poisons from the lung cavity. Psychiatrists today might point out that terrible deprivations in her life occasionally swept over her and left her lashing out at whoever was handy. And possibly she may have wondered if her husband, a handsome man in great demand by the ladies, had been faithful to her all her invalid years.

There is no way of knowing how it was between them after we children left and they were alone. Mother's letters to me were full of inconsequential chitchat, small jokes, newspaper clippings, snatches of songs she had liked, news of the dogs. Father's were large, generous scrawls, two- or three-sentence affairs enclosing a dollar bill for sodas and signed with his full name as if they were business letters.

This period must have been the best of all, for Mother was better, a semi-invalid but better. Still mindful of Dr. Brown's precepts, they began to travel, to Palm Beach, Miami, Havana, Nassau, on cruise ships to gentler climates where Saranac snows were like a cold and distant dream. Cruises were especially suitable, for a deck chair is the next thing to a cure chair if it is on the shady side. Consumptives were not allowed to stay in the sun.

It was a brave imitation of a normal life, a making-up for the years in Saranac. Mother would lie each morning on a reclining chair on the porch overlooking the resort golf course, the latest detective novel in hand, while my father, attired in white flannels and sporting a jaunty mustache, made his way around the links. After having rested all day, she could go to dinner at night, gamble at the tables, mind the stairs and watch the dancing. It was the best life yet since she had first clung to the bedpost and watched her own blood sink slowly into the rug.

"Get yourself a good chronic disease," Dr. Brown had said in parting. "Take good care of it and you'll outlive everyone else."

It was a joke, of course, he had meant it to be a small joke, and my mother had laughed because she knew it was expected. Privately, as she lay in the deck chair watching the gently undulating horizon, she turned it around and examined it closely, extracting the kernel of truth and comfort.

At home the garden was her delight, though she still avoided stairs and there were ten of them down the terrace bank to the garden. She took them carefully, but every day in the short summer season she took them, holding to the iron railing, carrying her basket and her scissors, wearing the floppy hat to guard against the sun. John, doubling as gardener, followed respectfully in her wake as she gathered armloads of peonies and roses, pointed out new plantings, places where plants must be staked. When I came home, she bribed me with pennies to dig the plantain weeds from the lawn and pick the pansies she could not stoop to pick herself.

The cellar of our house, with its steep stairs, remained forever as remote to her as the steppes of Siberia. The rows and rows of jams and jellies cooling on shelves in the storage room were something she could never see. Ironed laundry, muddy dogs, Mason jars full of the bounty of the surrounding fields emerged regularly from the cellar, but for seventeen years she knew it only as a door opening off the kitchen.

In my spare moments, when I was at home, I now took piano and bridge lessons, and I no longer talked like Nettie, the second maid who had been banished. Evenings when Mother was home we worked together on wooden jigsaw puzzles rented from the lending library in Utica. We spread them out on a card table, bending over them together, me consciously holding my breath when she leaned near to search for a particular piece. She was beautifully dressed and carefully marcelled, and when she leaned close, she smelled of L'Heure Bleu. But her breathing was audible and contained a strange rattle, and to this day the odor of L'Heure Bleu reminds me of my fear.

People were always coming to dinner, and the kitchen staff, who in those days took caste from the social position of their employers, gloried in the return to elegance my mother's arrival had brought. They hummed in the kitchen as they cut small bread rounds for canapés and whipped up elaborate desserts which my mother waved away. When the guests had repaired to the living room, the servants grilled me mercilessly about what had been said of the food. The town's supply cook, Molly O'Glollogie, widow of a Civil War veteran, went from house to house on party nights and knew, down to the last hors d'oeuvre, what had been served at the most recent parties in the homes of the others. Her coming was awaited with baited breath, and she always made the most of her moment, fending off questions while she removed her hat and tied on her apron, not divulging a word until they brought her a cup of steaming tea.

Mother's closet was full of dresses, all of which had been carefully chosen to hide her thin chest and arms. Sometimes she would pull one from the lot, glare at it angrily and declare that it made her look like a picked chicken. It would then be sent to the cleaner, altered to fit me in the sewing room and dispatched to be worn by me at the inevitable concert or piano recital with which our school weekends were filled. I never felt right about those gifts and kept them pushed to one side in the closet, alien butterflies in a closet stuffed with Peter Thompson uniform middies and skirts.

Mother and Father went to New York City often, and if it was a school holiday I went with them, wedged in between them behind John in the back seat. It was a long, tiring journey for an invalid, but driving was adjudged better by the doctors than the noise and inconvenience of the New York Central. Mother had always worn herself out in New York and she really shouldn't have gone, but New York was the mecca, the center of everything wonderful, and she continued to go. We took a picnic lunch no matter what the weather, having learned how to cope with cold in Saranac, and stopped at the first likely field when we got hungry, feasting on coffee and sandwiches atop a pile of buffalo robes. At the end of the day we drew up in front of the Algonquin Hotel, where I was booked into a room with my father and Mother slept alone. John stayed at the Royalton across the street, about which my father worried constantly because he considered the circular staircase a fire hazard.

Stern's was the only shop within striking distance for my

mother, and as soon as room service had cleared away breakfast, I would trail her through the arcade to 43rd Street, where for an hour or so I watched as she discarded invalidism in the excitement of Stern's hat department. She had a classic profile, the kind of straight-nosed, long-necked profile Gibson had made famous, and every hat was a temptation. The clerk there knew her and would greet her like a long-absent friend before disappearing to the rear to emerge later with armloads of plumed and befeathered and veiled creations, which Mother tried again and again while I amused myself with the rejects. When she had made a selection or two, we would walk back through the arcade, usually stopping for an early and ladylike lunch *à deux* at Alice Foote McDougall's.

And that was it. She had spent her strength until evening. She must rest the remainder of the day if she was to be able to go to the theater, which she loved. We invariably went, and afterward stopped for a drink in the lobby at a little table, sometimes with Frank Case, the hotel's owner, while I watched the resident cat come and go through his special door cut low near the kitchen.

"Where are the celebrities tonight, Frank?" my father would inquire, and Case would point out several here and there lifting a glass across the room.

My father always said afterward that he made them up, but neither my mother nor I believed it for a minute. Mother loved the Algonquin and its aura of fame.

I was closest to my mother in these moments, when I was a visitor at home and she was enjoying a standoff in her struggle against consumption. It was not an easy relationship. I think we were both trying too hard. We wanted to please each other. She consciously refrained from correcting or instructing me, and I, on my part, trailed her uncritically, not wanting to upset the balance of our friendship. We skimmed the surface of things that mattered, speaking of hats, of Fred Astaire, of the relative merits of fudge or marshmallow topping on ice cream, of Leslie Howard's last play. Privately I worried she was doing too much, that she would fall sick again and I would catch it, too.

I seldom saw my mother angry or depressed—we had too little time together to allow moods. We met on proper, polite terms. Once when we had been to the movies together, she whispered to me that we must go home at once, she had to go to the bathroom and hated cinema ladies' rooms. Later when she emerged from the bathroom at home, she said cheerfully that a bathroom when you need a bathroom is one of life's small pleasures.

I was immensely shocked. We were not on that footing. I had made her acquaintance too late in my growing up.

22 ❦

The Depression in our household was another subject, like
tuberculosis, that we did not mention. Or that was not, at
least, mentioned in my presence. I remember at school being
told to finish something on my plate because "there are plenty
who wish they had it." I was puzzled and inquired with
interest why—it was a particularly unappetizing piece of
haddock—and was informed that there was a Depression. It
was my first inkling.

I felt apologetic to have been so ignorant and innocent, but
there was no denying that was the way it was. The gradual
attrition of the household staff at home had puzzled me, but I
did not connect it with money. When I came home for

vacation, the trained nurse was gone, and I ceased to get letters from my parents with exotic postmarks, but these things meant nothing to me. Everything remained essentially the same. For me the Depression took place offstage, unmentioned and ignored.

It was only afterward I learned what my father had been going through. He had felt obliged to let John go, but since John had nowhere to go, he stayed on for his three meals a day. The Cadillac my father drove became more and more elderly—its upholstery had been chewed by an impatient waiting dog and hung in stalactites about my father's head from the car ceiling. His father was dead, and now it was he who sat at the old rolltop desk at the lumberyard. A delegation from the mill called on him to tell him they would take a small cut in pay if he would buy a new car. They understood the Mrs. was sick and expenses were heavy.

He refused, and when they had left he wept.

John continued to drive my mother, but he was searching in his spare time for paying work of any kind. The ancient Cadillac arrived to pick me up for a vacation driven by a strange man wearing a peaked cap and a lumber jacket. I allowed him to take my bag and stow it in the back of the car, but, while he was thus engaged, ran back into the school to tell the headmistress that a strange man was driving our car. In my mind I saw John bloody in the ditch, part of a plot to kidnap me, perhaps hold me for ransom. I sat quaking in my chair while she telephoned my father to learn that the usurper was his mill superintendent.

"Don't they tell you anything?" the poor man muttered, shoving the peaked cap back on his head as I climbed shamefaced in beside him.

John did not find paying work, and our household went

much as before, though now the staff seemed to be constantly changing. Sylvia, the current cook, disappeared; she was sick, they said; they had found another who was better. The food was indeed better, the kitchen ran smoother, I grew used to the new face. It was not until years later that my father told me that Sylvia had developed a cough, become convinced she had caught tuberculosis, and had sued my father for exposing her to the dangers of such an infectious disease. X-rays showed nothing, the suit was dismissed, but it was all added trauma. My mother stopped going into the kitchen for any reason.

I saw little of Mother. She was still an unfamiliar in my life, a figure sitting in the shadows in the back seat of the car, keeping out of the sun and watching from the window as I ran sweatily up and down a hockey field or took a horse over a jump. She would wave encouragingly to me through the window, smiling her dazzling smile. I think she was amused by the wholesome life in which I was immersed. Had she had the strength, there would have been no horses for her, no such nonsense; even I saw that in the way she smiled. It would have been shopping and theaters, some long walks to study the wild flowers about which she was always reading. But I think by now she had accepted the fact that she would have to make compromises all her life, that stairs and rest and milk would always loom large.

"I used to dream that I was dancing," she told my father once in my hearing, "doing the Charleston with everybody watching, clapping their hands, you know, because I was so good. Or maybe I was waltzing in a long, beautiful white dress. Not anymore. Now, even in my sleep I know I have tuberculosis.

A constant stream of little cardboard sputum envelopes,

tied carefully with tape and sealed, continued to find their way from our house to Dr. Brown's Saranac office, as meticulously wrapped as jewels lest the bacilli enclosed escape and contaminate some unsuspecting postal worker. The sputum was analyzed, and she returned regularly to Saranac for X-rays, but any reports she was given were announced out of my earshot. "How are the lake salamanders this season?" she inquired after a brief visit for a checkup. "I do think they look like small prehistoric dinosaurs." And, as an afterthought, "More X-rays. So boring."

I can see her still languidly sitting on our terrace, her thin legs crossed and the collie leaning against her knee. She is drinking a Manhattan cocktail before lunch and laughing at something my godmother is saying.

"Shall we get together for cards over the weekend?" asks my godmother. "Or does a day or so on the chaise longue sound better?"

"Cards, by all means," answers my mother, leaning to pick a burr from the collie's ear. "I am spoiling for a game."

For just a moment she seems like any of the other women who come to sit on the terrace, lunch when my father is in New York City, chattering about their gardens and their children. But now it is early afternoon, the meal has been eaten, the guest gone and it is time for her rest. I have gone upstairs to find something in my room and on the way down come upon her unexpectedly, the eternal glass of milk in her hand, stopping to rest as always on the landing.

She rearranges her face when she catches sight of me, wipes it clean of everything, giving me a bright smile and resuming the upward journey. But I have seen the bleak, lost look of someone who briefly considers that things may never improve. It is an image that has stayed with me all these years.

She came to my graduation, sitting demurely beside my father in her picture hat, craning her neck to see how my dress hung and measuring with a critical eye my classmates in their turn marching up the aisle. It amused her to find that, because my friends' names changed so often with the marital status of their mothers, I stumbled on the introduction even of my roommate. But she put them all at ease—perched on my bed to direct my packing, admiring their yearbook inscriptions, selecting records for the little wind-up portable victrola while I packed the flotsam and jetsam of my six years' stay.

I was immensely proud of her. I was seventeen and no longer uneasy in her presence. We were both women of the world.

That summer my father rented a small camp on a nearby lake within easy driving distance, where my mother and I spent long afternoons feeding a family of chipmunks from our fingers and staring out at the water dotted with little sailboats. Mother loved that camp, which belonged to a friend who had built it with the proceeds of a lucky gambling streak in Nassau. She loved the hours we spent there sitting in deck chairs as she sketched the view, Gibson Girls with pompadours or the collie lying at her feet. I gathered armloads of wild flowers and filled the camp with jars of them, did crossword puzzles while she sewed name tapes on my sweaters and coats. I was going to college in the fall.

If John was busy, she drove the car that brought us there. It was her car and her life—I was only spending a few weeks in her company. I think now it took a good deal out of her, and that she knew it and consciously chose to do it anyway, but it did not cross my mind then. My life lay elsewhere, in a dozen other cities where I had made my friends. She must have known this. It must have made her a little sad, but it was she who had arranged it that way.

She wasn't sleeping well.

"I couldn't sleep last night," she said to my father over the dinner table. "I came in from the sleeping porch and tried the bed in my room. It had nerves in it, too."

My father looked up in alarm.

"It was only that I couldn't sleep," she explained patiently, studying her ring. "It happens."

He made sympathetic clucking noises.

"It doesn't matter," she said. "I shouldn't have told you. Nothing matters if you can get up out of the bed. I remember about that."

"Eat your meat, Betty," said my father to me as if I were again ten years old.

It was my seventeenth summer. I should have been used to the way things were in our house, but I still lived in the shadow of the fear. Each morning when I heard my mother coughing, I lay in my bed, the muscles in my stomach tightening, wondering if I, too, might some morning wake to find I had a deep cough with a frightening catch in it, a cough that reached to the bottom of my lungs. I had been away so long I had forgotten the sound of it. I resolved to eat more sensibly, not to stay out too late, to be more careful. Tuberculosis struck like a thug in a dark alley, without warning; I knew that. Possibly I was even now carrying the bacilli in my lungs.

My parents had long since ceased to warn me to be careful, for our precautions were now routine, a way of life never to be deviated from. Still, though I was ashamed to be, I was scarred with the fear. It lay in the back of my mind, like an unruly black dog waiting to jump when I wasn't watching, whenever something reminded me of the symptoms, the uncertainty, the possibility. I remembered my brother lying in the cure chair, turning the pages of his book with his mittened hands, and I felt the brackish taste of the hemorrhaging blood in my own mouth.

I was ashamed of my feelings, but I was not unhappy when it was time to leave for college.

❦ 23

I think my mother knew she was dying then, before I went off to college the first year. I have watched people I love die since then and I am convinced that victims of the two dread diseases, tuberculosis and cancer, know when the fight becomes too uneven, when they struggle in too deep a bog in spite of all the bright and encouraging words of family and doctors. I think there comes a time in a terminal disease when the ill unplug themselves from life, detach their minds—when they look inward and see that it is time to let go.

Dickens, who lived in a time that knew TB intimately, spoke of this. Tuberculosis, he said, "is a dread disease in which the struggle between soul and body is so gradual, quiet and solemn, and the result so sure, that day by day, and grain by grain, the mortal past wastes and withers away. . . ."

I don't know when my mother knew the struggle was too much. She wasn't one for solemn moments. The old medical histories of TB refer often to the burst of activity which precedes the end, and I think it was that way with her. I was, as usual, unaware of what was going on at the time. If I thought anything, it was that my mother was better, but perhaps that was only because we had finally reached a plateau of mutual, easy cordiality.

She came to see me with my father at college that first year. They stayed nearby in Amherst at the Lord Jeff, of which she became enamored. She loved the little New England village square, the student who came in after dinner to play show tunes in exchange for his meal, the deep old fireplace you could sit in.

It was a rather difficult weekend because John had taken the car with him when he went to his rooming house at night and parked it in the side yard. During the night the house caught fire, burned all his clothing and badly singed the side of the Cadillac. John had to spend the rest of the weekend dressed in my father's clothes, which made Mother giggle. She said he looked like Charlie Chaplin.

She seemed especially gay that weekend. She did not try to conceal her amusement at the white angora ankle socks and tennis shoes I was wearing in subzero February weather, much the style on campus, but she made amends by offering to knit me a new pair. She took an interest in my courses and what I thought about everything. She was reading Hemingway and was anxious to know how I felt about him. She inspected my room and said she would send a new bedspread.

I thought she looked wonderful. She was wearing a beautiful aqua rabbit's-hair wool dress with a V neck which she had filled in with several strands of beads. "It has such a wretchedly low neckline," she said, making a little moue of distaste. "It makes me look scrawny, but the color *is* heavenly, don't you think?"

That summer I brought seven Smith freshmen back with me to stay for a week in our little camp on the lake. Mother dutifully wrote each of their mothers making the invitation official, packed her bags and fled the scene in the car behind John, heading for the Lord Jeff, where she stayed until everyone was gone. I gave it no thought at the time. Neither I nor any of my friends had ever been drunk, and we were planning to rectify that omission. We were busy making plans to buy a bottle of gin, elect one of us to remain sober to report, and drink until we reached that loose state of inebriation we had so often watched in our escorts. We never found out what it was like, for we laid by only a pint for the experiment, but it was all very absorbing.

Late in the summer Mother returned to Saranac for pneumothorax, a procedure in which gas is introduced into the chest wall to force the diseased lung to collapse and thus rest. It was an exceedingly traumatic operation, for, like all surgery for consumptives, it had to be done with the patient fully conscious.

In the operation a long needle was inserted between the ribs to pierce the chest wall. The sound was one of the worst things about it—rather like a knitting needle going through heavy cardboard. Patients who had undergone pneumothorax often suffered noisy breathing afterwards, whistling like ancient draft horses pulling uphill. But the operation was much the fashion in the late thirties. Folklore has it that a Canadian doctor in Saranac once administered pneumothorax to himself, having been refused it by his doctor as unsuitable in his case. Irving Altman still has pneumothorax every three months; the gas dissipates and must be renewed frequently. Only one doctor in Saranac still uses the technique.

I don't know if it gave my mother even temporary respite. I went back to college, unaware, assuming that the world on Maple Street would continue as it always had, with Mother living the sort of half-life to which we had all grown used.

When I came home at Christmas my father met me at the station alone. He seemed suddenly older than I had remembered and my mother thinner. There was a new rug in her room and a cabinet radio by her chaise longue. She was working a needlepoint chair seat for the first of eight chairs in the dining room and she was through all but the right-hand corner. I thought she seemed engrossed but a little distracted, as I perched in the little chintz-covered chair.

"I didn't see John," I said.

She put down the needlepoint and began to fiddle with the coffee cup on the table beside her.

"I hate it to be me who tells you," she said after a minute, "and I think now we were wrong not to have told you when it happened. John is gone. He died four days ago. Something to do with being gassed in the war. You know he'd had pneumonia. His lungs were bad. We buried him in the family plot along with everyone else. Just yesterday."

She looked up at last, ceasing to avoid my eye.

"I'm sorry, darling," she said.

I felt bereft, betrayed and angry, and the lump in my throat threatened to strangle me.

"I'm sorry," she said again, and now she was looking over my shoulder at the snow drifting lazily down on the hemlocks outside, a little as if she weren't paying attention. "We thought we'd wait to tell you, as long as you were coming so soon. There was nothing you could have done, and you were coming so soon."

"I would have liked to have been there," I said and stumbled out of the room somehow, stiff with resentment.

"There was nothing you could have done, darling," Mother called once more after my retreating back. "We loved him, you know."

I didn't cry until that night, alone, in bed.

I am amazed now how unperceptive I was, how little I was aware that she would not be completing eight dining-room chair seats. *Pas devant les enfants,* up to the grave itself. There was nothing I could do.

I was back at college, and the letters from home gave no hint how bad things were. I think they were considering thorocoplasty, the last-resort operation, but for some reason they discarded the idea. Perhaps the doctors recommended against it, perhaps Mother herself chose not to go through this grueling procedure. She had known many in Saranac who had submitted to it, and was well aware what was involved.

Thorocoplasty was hard even on the doctors—a long, long operation which was a terrible shock to the patient. Of course it had to be done under local anesthetic, so the patient missed nothing of what was going on. It was usually done in three stages because it was so demanding of both patient and doctor.

A long incision was made down the back a few inches from the backbone. The physician then removed nine ribs in order to collapse the lung permanently. Often the infection spilled from the bad lung into the good because the patient was forced to lie on his side during the operation. The sound of rib removal was enormously loud in the operating room, and the fully conscious patient suffered unbelievable mental anguish.

The procedure generally left the patient with a severely crippled hand, and for some reason this condition was apparently worse in women. It was necessary to do exercises for a long time to bring function back into clawlike fingers. A layer of cartilage gradually built up to take the place of the ribs, but the body remained somewhat concave. Not too long ago, in Saranac, a man who had had thorocoplasty died in an automobile accident. An autopsy was ordered, but the presiding pathologist discovered it was impossible to break the layer of cartilage over his lung even with a hammer. They knew at once what his history was.

Mother decided against this operation, if indeed she ever gave it any serious consideration. In February I received a telephone call from Father suggesting I come home for the weekend. Nothing was wrong, only they were a little lonesome.

To my blind eyes, everything seemed the same.

"Is it all right, the school?" she asked me with unaccustomed directness, making a great business of lighting up a cigarette.

Fine, I told her.

"And the piano? How is it going? You fudge with the left hand, you know."

I promised to do better. She told me she was rereading *Pickwick Papers.* How long since I had read it?

We had a steak dinner which she managed to conceal under her knife. I thought she seemed withdrawn, possibly tired. She talked desultorily of how the chair seats would improve the dining room and what the snow had done to the apple tree. But mostly she let me chatter on.

The last time I saw her she was lying in her chaise longue in her negligee, staring speculatively at the needlepoint. She didn't think she would come to the station to see me off. I wouldn't mind, would I?

When I bent to brush her cheek with mine, the arm she put about me was as light as a moth's wing.

"Stand up straight, darling," she said, patting my cheek.

I never saw her alive again.

24 ❧

I can't remember how I heard the news of my mother's death. Someone must have handed me a message to call home— someone, somewhere—but I don't remember the moment. I remember only a long train ride toward home in the dark, sitting alone in the coach car, changing tracks at Albany, standing stunned in the cold dark while the New York Central rearranged its cars. To the very last I had had no warning of what was to happen.

When I got off the train at the depot, my father was waiting for me alone. His kiss on my cheek was icy cold, but his free hand groped for mine.

"Well, she's gone," was all he said.

We went down the marble steps she had so often hurried up to meet him, and we were still holding hands. I couldn't bring myself to ask for any details, and he seemed lost in his thoughts. We drove home in the ancient Cadillac almost in silence.

It was in the time before funeral parlors took death into their anterooms, and Mother lay in her own bed in her bedroom as if she were simply asleep. We stood, Father and I—where was my brother?—by the fireplace at the end of the room, not really looking at her but unwilling to leave her alone. She looked the same, but remote, carved in stone.

"I couldn't save her," said my heartbroken father as much to me as anyone, and for the first time I felt the delicate balance between us shift. He was leaning on me, his child, for comfort.

I told him he had managed to extend her life seventeen years longer than it might otherwise have been, but he had forgotten me again. He was looking at her.

"I did everything I could, Bess," he said softly, as if she could hear him and absolve him of any blame, and once more I felt like an intruder between them.

When he turned away for the last time, I told him again that he had managed to extend her life, but he only shook his head. I hope I was telling him the truth, that what he did for her made a difference.

There is no way of knowing.

It was a small-town funeral. When I got up the next morning, my mother's friends were sitting in every chair of the living room, dressed in black and ramrod straight, ready to answer the phone, receive visitors, lend support wherever they were needed. The room was already full of the sweet, moist, hothouse smell of flowers, and a silver pot of coffee sat on the table.

In the kitchen the staff was dissolved in tears, feeling none of the compulsion felt in the living room to bear up. They went about their duties red-eyed, weeping into the dishwater, sobbing occasionally.

There was no place anywhere for me.

I went through the kitchen into the cold room, an anteroom where once the wooden icebox had stood and which was now shut off and used for storage. Beyond the walls of the little room I could hear the household going about its business. I pressed my forehead against the cold glass of the one little window overlooking the driveway, and at last I cried for my mother.

Through my tears I stared at the snowbanks lining the driveway while the servants moved about the kitchen, and I knew I was crying not for the loss of my mother but because I had never really known her. She and my father had made a life together in spite of tuberculosis, but in any true love affair there are casualties, and I was one of them.

After a while I wiped away the tears and went back into the kitchen. They were busy with the roasts and pies that must be cooked on an occasion like this, the coffee to be made, the salads to be mixed. People would be coming and going; the house was already full. I felt like an intruder, a stranger in my own house with nothing at all to do. It was all being taken care of without me. I went upstairs and sat on my bed alone, trying to get used to the idea that Mother was dead.

The undertaker, who was also the coroner, arrived and went upstairs with my father and Pearl, the pretty young second maid. When they came down together, my mother's diamond engagement ring was in Pearl's apron pocket. "Give it to Betty," said my father, and she reached deep into the starchy apron pocket and extended it to me on the flat of her hand. I looked at it a long time and then I put it on my finger. It was the first time I really accepted the fact that my mother was gone.

A day or two later we sat upstairs in my father's bedroom while the funeral guests gathered, all three of us in a row on the bed as the icy drafts from the opening front door crept up the stairs with every arriving mourner. Mother lay in her coffin in the front parlor, and after a while we heard the murmur of the minister's voice begin: "I am the resurrection and the life. . . ."

We buried her in the family plot, not too far from where John lay and close by the plot reserved for my father. I hoped John would be wherever she was to take care of her. My brother, remembering things of which my father and I could have no knowledge, looked on impassively as they lowered her into the earth. And then it was all over, and I went back to college, leaving my father alone in the big house.

Every age seems innocent to the one that follows it, but my parents now seem to me singularly unequipped to have dealt with what happened to them. A pretty small-town belle and a young man whose grandfather had long ago ensured his comfortable future, they might have been characters from a Fitzgerald novel who blundered by chance into a Dostoevskian drama. They dwelt in a small, safe, pleasant world in which they had had every expectation of remaining. They seemed wrong for tragedy.

How did they manage—they with their Abercrombie & Fitch fishing rods, their ivory-faced Mah-Jongg sets and their kitchen full of servants—to cope with the inescapable reality of tuberculosis for half a lifetime? Without any weapons against such an overpowering illness, without Blue Cross to pay the bills, without a psychiatrist to assure them they had intolerable burdens and were entitled to trauma, how did they manage not to be beaten down in the long, uneven fight?

It was all foreshadowed in the letters lying in the little doll's trunk. "Lay aside all care and worry and come back from Florida strong and completely rested," writes my mother's father to his Dearest Little Daughter on her honeymoon. "Tell Ted to make you keep up your diet of eggs," pleads her brother, Frank. "Darling Jim, take care." Why did he call her Jim? It is all gone forever with them.

For much of their life together my mother was an exile and my father alone, but they managed to make a life. There was, after all, nothing else to do, and the less said about it, the better. They lived in a time which feared even a whisper of the disease from which she suffered. Things were difficult, but it was, they knew, a brave new age. Each generation breaks its own new ground. In the house in which my father was brought up, the newspaper was stitched up the middle and warmed before his parents read it.

They would cope. They had the very best doctors, they had Saranac, if there was a cure, they would find it.

"Don't come too near your mother," my father said to me all my life, and of course I never did. I leaned away from her when she stooped to pin my hem for my piano recital, frightened by the sound of the rattle in her lungs. I held my breath when she pointed over my shoulder at the wrong word in the crossword puzzle, refused the piece of candy she handed me from her fingers.

"I never did that before," she said, looking at me, blue eyes wide with surprise at her own temerity. "But I just washed my hands."

I only shook my head and drew away. No soap and water could wash away tuberculosis. I knew that. I was imprinted with the fear, she did not know how to reach across it, and when she died we were still only polite friends.

Years later, when I was going through her things, I came across the little silver card case she carried to parties. She was a great one for tucking away the words to songs in odd places—in books, under the clock, in the pockets of her dresses—and here was another, yellowing with age in the stiff leather compartment of the case where the cards had once been.

I lifted it out carefully and laid it out on the table, piecing together the places where the paper was ripped. It was the old Negro spiritual "Child, I know you're going to miss me when I'm gone."

Kafka, who suffered from TB himself, called the disease "the germ of death itself, intensified." A disease of the lungs, says Susan Sontag, is metaphorically a disease of life. There are enough people living today who remember TB so that when an ancient cemetery where victims of the disease lay was dug up to move it from the path of development, there was public outcry that the old graves were still too dangerous to open.

Tuberculosis may have been the first of the pestilences, but a whole generation has grown up which has scarcely heard of the white plague. In 1976 there were 32,000 new cases of tuberculosis reported, but it was hardly remarked. Since the advent of drug therapy, a diagnosis of TB is an inconvenience only. Within weeks a new case is non-infectious and the patient returns to his job, his home and his life without losing the rhythms of his world. He may have to take drugs for two years, but even that is changing. Soon, they say, drug therapy will be reduced to six months.

"They used to tell us they were going to put us to bed for

three weeks when they diagnosed TB," says Irving Altman. "You could stand that. You couldn't have stood it if you'd known it was for years."

In my dreams I go back to that house where we all lived, wandering about it in my unconscious as if nothing at all had changed. And sometimes I stand again in that cold bedroom where Mother lies dead after the long struggle.

"I couldn't save her," my father, dead himself a quarter-century, says once more in my ear, and in my dream I shut my eyes against the remembered look on his face.

We did what we could, I tell him silently as I did on the day she died, but in my dream I turn away and beg her, wherever she is, to forgive me.